THE CUTTING EDGE OF COMPASSION

PRAISE

"With the recent changes in the American medical system, both doctors and patients are experiencing a degree of frustration. So how can physicians and the people they have committed to treating work through the morass of insurance, ethics, the legal system and basic human decency to create a system which works for everyone? In this book, Dr. Barry Rose lays out a simple, common-sense and compassionate approach which anyone concerned with medicine would do well to read."

- Joel Comm, *New York Times* Best-Selling Author

"Cutting edge and compassion are not words often used in the same sentence but are desperately needed. Thank you, Barry Rose for writing a dynamic new book that offers innovative thinking, a fresh mindset and solid tools that will positively impact every area of life."

- Marcia Wieder, CEO, Dream University and Founder, The Meaning Institute

"Elegantly written in the first person, this book offers us a story both highly personal and profoundly universal. Writing in the first person and using his own life experience as a parable, Dr. Barry Rose clarifies some the core principles of the ancient lineage of medicine and demonstrates their relevance to the world of today. *The Cutting Edge of Compassion* offers a potent prescription not only for the healing of our health care system but the healing of our society itself. This book is a must read for anyone considering a future in medicine and for anyone, no matter what profession they have chosen to follow, who wishes to make of their own lives a blessing and a work of healing."

- Rachel Naomi Remen, M.D., *New York Times* Best-Selling Author, *Kitchen Table Wisdom* and *My Grandfather's Blessings*

"A classic American success story showing the importance of persistence and mentoring."

- Byron J. Masterson, M. D. FACS, FACOG, J. Wayne Reitz Professor of Obstetrics and Gynecology, Emeritus, University of Florida, Gainesville, Florida

THE CUTTING EDGE OF COMPASSION

*How Physicians, Health Professionals, and Patients Can
Build Healing Relationships Based on Trust*

BARRY ROSE, M.D.

NEW YORK

The Cutting Edge of Compassion
How Physicians, Health Professionals, and Patients Can Build
Healing Relationships Based on Trust

Published in New York, New York, by Morgan James Publishing. Morgan James and The Entrepreneurial Publisher are trademarks of Morgan James, LLC. www.MorganJamesPublishing.com

The Morgan James Speakers Group can bring authors to your live event. For more information or to book an event visit The Morgan James Speakers Group at www.TheMorganJamesSpeakersGroup.com.

9781630477806   paperback
9781630477813   eBook
9781630477820   hardcover

Library of Congress Control Number: 2015914792

Shelfie

A **free** eBook edition is available with the purchase of this print book.

CLEARLY PRINT YOUR NAME ABOVE IN UPPER CASE

Instructions to claim your free eBook edition:
1. Download the Shelfie app for Android or iOS
2. Write your name in **UPPER CASE** above
3. Use the Shelfie app to submit a photo
4. Download your eBook to any device

Cover Design by:
Chris Treccani
chris@3dogdesign.net

Interior Design by:
Brittany Bondar

In an effort to support local communities, raise awareness and funds, Morgan James Publishing donates a percentage of all book sales for the life of each book to Habitat for Humanity Peninsula and Greater Williamsburg.

Get involved today! Visit
www.MorganJamesBuilds.com

Habitat
for Humanity®
Peninsula and
Greater Williamsburg
Building Partner

In memory of Ruth Rose

CONTENTS

INTRODUCTION: IN THE BEGINNING

Love and compassion are necessities, not luxuries.
Without them humanity cannot survive.

Dalai Lama

My first memorable experience with a physician occurred at the age of five. In the 1950s, before the days of seatbelts and color TV, it wasn't uncommon for children to ride around in cars standing on the seats, enjoying the scenery. One day, my cousin and I were doing just that—standing in the front passenger seat while my aunt was driving. Suddenly, my aunt hit the brakes, trying to avoid a car that had pulled out in front of her. She instinctively stuck out her right arm, trying to protect us from falling forward. Fortunately, she caught my cousin, but her arm wasn't long enough to catch me. Into the dashboard I propelled, catching most of the blow just above my right eye.

My next recollection was lying on a table with a light shining like the sun into my eye, blinding me as I looked up through a red, foggy blur. I kept reaching up to block the light with my hand, until finally my arms were restrained, as the doctor sutured my eyelid. I don't recall any pain, but the fear was so profound that for many years afterwards, and still occasionally to this day, I woke up in a cold sweat, reaching up to block that bright light burning into my dreams.

With an introduction like this, why would I ever choose medicine as a profession? None of my family members had anything to do with medicine or healing the sick. My mother was an Avon lady, wandering from door to door, peddling lipsticks and nail polish (like the mother in the movie *Edward Scissorhands*), and my father was a traveling chemical salesman.

One week, when my father was in town, he took me to the emergency room after I had cut my hand on a broken window. I remember that the wound was burning and gaped open, oozing redness, but the bleeding was easily controlled with direct pressure. I was taken to a small exam room with a movable overhead light, and a nurse proceeded to scrub my hand with brown soapy fluid. Soon afterwards, in walked a doctor with scraggy, curly brown hair, wearing greens and a white coat. He told me that he was going to numb my wound and sew up the laceration. At about that time, my father started to swoon as the blood drained from his face, and a nurse had to escort him to the waiting room before he passed out and hit the floor. I was left alone to face the drama ahead.

As I gritted my teeth, watching the doc fill up the syringe with lidocaine from a little rubber-capped bottle, I braced for the pain. As he started numbing my wound with small punctures into my open cut, I felt some burning but, surprisingly, no pain. I curiously watched as he sutured my wound with simple stitches, one after another. He was totally absorbed in this process, neatly tying his knots. When he finished, he said, "Well, I'm done—looks like nine stitches." I immediately responded, "No, there's ten." He turned and looked at me, surprised that I actually had been watching while he was absorbed in the task at hand. He counted again and said, "You're right." I beamed, feeling like I had been an active part of my procedure. I was intrigued by the experience, and looking back, it may have been the earliest sign that I thought this medicine thing was something cool. Many years later, another sign would come.

It's a mystery sometimes how people gravitate towards their role in life. What makes someone want to be a doctor, a nurse, an accountant, or an architect? Many times people are guided by their strengths and natural aptitudes. A person who is great with numbers might be led towards the path of being an accountant or a banker, for example. Others seem to just "know" what they are meant to be and discover their passions early in life. Still others have many gifts and talents and may change careers multiple times on their quest to find what satisfies their core interests.

As for me, I know that when I was a sixth grader, sitting in Mr. Miller's science class studying the human body, something within me changed. At the age of twelve, I should have simply been satisfied with focusing on baseball and girls. But I was fascinated with the muscles of the body and the bones of the skeleton. I found myself on a quest for knowledge about this new medical world. A decade later, when I was applying to medical school, I contacted my beloved sixth-grade teacher Mr. Miller to ask him, with gratitude, to write me a letter of recommendation. And so my journey as a healer began and continues to present day. It's been an extraordinary path that has led me to practice and experience compassionate healing.

I have worked in a number of different practice settings, but to date, the most enjoyable has been my present practice. I am the chief of orthopedics and the surgical division head for the Alameda division of the Palo Alto Medical Foundation headquartered in Palo Alto, California. It is one of the top-ten largest multi-specialty groups in California. Its level of care is exemplary and a model of what is possible in great medical care.

I am not a writer, just a guy from Kansas who became a doctor and then an orthopedic surgeon. However, it's time to share what I've learned along the way. Don't be surprised if I enroll you in my passion.

In this book, I don't offer an evidence-based, authoritative diagnosis of the healthcare system. Instead, I share my stories, because every physician finds his or her own path to medicine. For some, it is a calling, a vocation, even a destiny. For others, it is a legacy; it's is in their DNA. In part 1, I share my own story about being called into medicine, and in the telling of my story, I hope other physicians may discover their story, too.

However, my story is part of a bigger story—one that includes physicians, health professionals, and patients. Naturally, taking care of the sick and injured has many challenges. As physicians, our primary job is to find the root cause of an illness or injury and then use all of our tools, as well as the insights of our patients, to affect positive change. We have to discern what we can change or heal, and what we cannot. I have often wondered if we could come up with a definitive, step-by-step guide for success in our clinical practice as physicians—perhaps like the DSM-V for psychologists. I have often traveled down a treatment path that led to heartache instead of hope, when my efforts did not produce a satisfactory result. Yet, I always learn much from the process.

If healing and helping is an intuitive process that develops with age and experience, then the guidebook is already within us. I believe that coming from a place of integrity and trusting your gut is the best guide for all of us as healers, in any circumstance. Truly understanding our patients and their personality types will help in the process. We also have amazing diagnostic tools, like MRIs, laboratory tests, and scans that complement and test our intuition.

Yet in recent years, both physicians and patients have noticed a shift from trust to suspicion in Western medicine and other healing arts. As we'll see in part 2, I believe the physician/patient relationship is the first step in the healing that needs to takes place for improved outcomes.

Healthcare practitioners undergo exhaustive training for years and usually at a sacrifice. But patients also have a responsibility for their own care and well-being. True healing starts with the patient and his or her care provider working together as a team. Mutual respect is important. Everyone— patients, physicians, and other healthcare professionals—needs to appreciate each other's gifts and understand how they can affect care.

The healthcare industry is not just composed of physicians, allied health professionals, and patients, however. Fear, ego, and greed have also entered healthcare through the insurance industry, the legal system, and the pharmaceutical industry. As a surgeon, I definitely love to fix things in need of repair and afterwards get to experience the joy of someone regaining his or her health and mobility in a short period of time. I feel the same way about our healthcare system. I have seen healthcare change significantly since I graduated from medical school in 1979. Back then, just being a doctor granted you great respect. Hospitals catered to us, and patients rarely questioned us. I don't remember out-of-control medication costs or insurance companies in denial about these costs—though I do remember a big fear of being sued, with little tort reform or caps on punitive damages.

I know many physicians, healers, holistic practitioners following Eastern philosophies, and patients alike who have voiced their desire for a change in medicine and a better way to heal. Together, we can figure out the best way for all of us to get well. Yes, there are many obstacles to overcome, considering our intractable legal, insurance, and pharmaceutical systems, but together, I feel we can make transformations that afford us better, happier, and healthier lives. Trust is paramount.

So in this book, I hope to lead us all—patients and healers of all kinds—away from fear, ego, and greed and toward a place of trust and compassion in healthcare. Being in a state of stress and fear knocks down our immune system and keeps all of us from healing. I want to share with you steps physicians and other healthcare practitioners need to take, followed by suggestions for patients to engage in for their healing and, finally, what the system needs to do to take us from fear to compassion, trust, and healing.

At the end, I hope we will have a vision for what compassionate healthcare can be and how we can all work together to make this happen. I hope I can sign you up to take on this challenge with me. I can't do it alone, but we certainly can do it together. I hope that when you read my thoughts, not only will you have a better understanding of who each of us are, but also what all of us truly need. It's time for us to make changes to our healthcare system that will afford us the best possible life to enjoy in the short time that we live on this planet.

PART ONE

Called to Care

My mission in life is not merely to survive, but to thrive; and to do so with some passion, some compassion, some humor, and some style.

Maya Angelou

1. THE RESPONSIBILITY

When you inherit a broken family, you can't throw it away and get a new one. What you can do is find people and situations that provide for you what your family cannot.

Iyanla Vanzant

When an adolescent gets thrown into the deep end, with water over his head, he either sinks or swims. At least, that's what it felt like when I was faced, time after time, with the responsibility of keeping my family together. Growing up with an alcoholic parent had profound effects on all of us.

I'm not sure when I first realized my mom had a drinking problem. She was always sweet and loving and extremely close with her mother. My father traveled as a salesman and was gone from Monday through Friday, so my mom's emotional support came from my grandmother. My grandmother was always in our home and vice versa. When I was thirteen, my grandmother was diagnosed with leukemia. She had been tired for months, and once diagnosed, she dwindled quickly and died three months later. My mom was devastated. Her best friend was gone, and my father could not provide the support she needed. This loss was too much for my mom to endure. My mom, the bright, sweet, high school valedictorian, needed to escape on a daily basis. So she dove into a bottle, and I took it upon myself to try to keep her from drowning. This sense of family responsibility at an early age would eventually evolve into my journey toward becoming a healer.

Every day at around four o'clock, my mother would start to drink. She drank openly at first, but later, as my father chided her, she became more secretive. Yet the results were always the same. She did her best to get dinner on the table for my brother and me, and then she would fade to black. She wandered around, out of it, and then would pass out on the bed, usually before my little brother and I would go to sleep. At first, I was filled with fear over what to do. That unsettling, gut-wrenching feeling I got when my mother would slur her words and could barely communicate became commonplace. I can remember times when I couldn't arouse her and worried she was dead. I had to console my brother's tears as he watched her stupor. My dad was on the road, so I was the only one in charge. I inherited the role of parental caretaker long before my time, but somebody had to do it. It was hard for a thirteen-year-old. The drama became the norm.

In the morning, my mom was apologetic and filled with guilt on a regular basis. She would become overly attentive to us and smothered us with loving gestures. She would cook us French toast and sausage for breakfast to try to make up for the night before.

At some point, she admitted she had a problem. But my "responsible" dad, who traveled to produce an income for his family, left the responsibility of taking care of his wife to his teenage son. I was supposed to mark the liquor bottles for him while he was traveling. When he came home on the weekends, he would check those bottles. If the alcohol level had dropped below the mark from the week before, all hell would break loose. He would then beat her up emotionally when he inevitably discovered she'd been drinking. He would yell and scream at her and my "scapegoat" brother, further escalating the drama. I was spared because I was the "family pleaser," a well-established role in a typical alcoholic family. I doubt if my father ever understood that it wasn't an appropriate role for me.

I can still remember many times when my dad would yell at my mother while taking his belt off in response to my smart-ass brother. We suffered through meals where my mom would silently serve us after one of my dad's outbursts, and my brother and I would eat with our heads down, afraid to look up. The shame was often overwhelming.

Yet my role sometimes had positive results. When the family was in total disorder, I stepped in. In all the chaos, I would sometimes make everyone sit down to have a family meeting. My dad couldn't turn on me because I was his little scout and carried out his requests. At the same time, my mother and brother depended on me for their caretaking and emotional support. At age sixteen, I was keeping the family together. What power I had as a teenager! My life was like James Taylor's song "Fire and Rain." My father was the fire, and I was the rain that put it out. Sadly, we kept up the appearance of a normal family to both our extended family and our friends, following an unspoken rule never to talk about what happened at home behind closed doors.

When I turned seventeen, I worked for my dad in his own chemical company. He and his partner had developed allergies to the toxic chemicals, so he had me mixing them. Just as before, he didn't consider that perhaps it wasn't good for me to be exposed to the toxicity either. That kind of disconnect was typical. It has taken me decades finally to let go of trying to squelch the uncontrollable energy force that my father represents. My mother, much later in her sobriety, tried to bring him back to a place of normalcy. I'm afraid the stress she dealt with as well as her strong family history of cancer, cost her dearly and added to her early demise, helping to bring on and accelerate her cancer. To this day, I finally feel I have a handle on how to deal with his crazymaking behavior.

Yet in his own way, I feel my father did the best job he could. The only thing I have power over is my own energy, and I can choose to stay positive and avoid the negative, which helps restore my soul and my sanity. I had to learn how to balance my life as a result of my imposed responsibility, and learn I did. Through my upbringing, I learned some great life lessons, even though many times I was burned from the fire.

That said, unhealthy caretaking creates emotional baggage that can become too much to bear alone. For a brief time during my medical training, I lived with my brother as he finished graduate school. He was in the middle of dealing with his revelation of being gay and presenting it to my family and the world around him. The combination of clinics, my mother's alcoholism, my father's abdication of his responsibility, and my brother's issues with substance abuse and sexuality became too much to handle.

My brother came home one day and, after searching the apartment, found me curled up in the fetal position inside a dark bedroom closet, barely responsive. To this day, I truly don't remember it. Apparently I had completely separated from reality as some kind of escape mechanism. Looking back, I believe it was the beginning of my process of separating from unhealthy caretaking and focusing my energy on situations I could affect positively.

I can still remember seeing a therapist, decades ago, about the effects my family's alcoholism had on me and how to cope with all the guilt and codependence. I was astounded at how I fit the typical role of "family pleaser" in my family unit. I have a much greater understanding now than I did then about the genetic predisposition to conditions like alcoholism and cystic fibrosis. My mother and her brother, as well as their parents, were all dependent on alcohol. Of the four sons my mother and her brother had between them, I was the only one without the gene for alcoholism or drug dependency—yet I have a son with similar issues.

The role of the health professional most certainly involves taking care of others. It requires compassion and empathy. It also requires a sense of responsibility and integrity to do whatever is needed to assist in someone's care. We have a huge job when directing the care of others. We are the experts, and if we don't do our job well, the patient will suffer the most. Our skill in this role develops with time and experience. It also has to do with one's inherent nature. The caring I feel for others comes from a place of very positive energy and love. Occasionally, the role of caretaker is bestowed upon you as a result of necessity at an early age, as it was for me. Although it was initially unpleasant and inappropriate, it propelled me toward a life's mission for caring that exists to this day. My caretaking role began with my mother, father, and brother, and as time went on, it extended to my children and ultimately to my patients. I hope that my sense of responsibility for caretaking has been refined and channeled to a more appropriate and less codependent role. My early experiences, although at times very painful, strengthened me and have allowed me to rise to meet some difficult challenges, both in medicine and in life. My biggest lesson is learning that the cornerstone of compassion is forgiveness. I was able to forgive my parents completely from that which consumed me during my earlier years. This has helped me become a better physician.

Ultimately, caregivers need to have compassion for themselves before they can be truly compassionate with their patients. If you are a physician, I invite you to remember your journey to healing and the sacrifices you have made along the way. Rediscovering your primary motivation for becoming a healer in the first place is the best way to stay on the path of integrity and compassion when helping those you care for.

2. THE INFLUENCE

To be kind is more important than to be right.
Many times what people need is not a brilliant
mind that speaks but a special heart that listens.
And it is compassion that makes a special heart
move to the pain of others. Be a compassionate and
loving human being.

Rishika Jain

I have often wondered what it is that draws one to the world of healing. Is it a fix-it mentality or an aura of pure caring? Does it come from a place of ego, power, and control? Maybe it includes all these motivations, at least in part. Many times we can identify someone or something that has influenced and motivated us to pursue a specific career choice.

In tenth grade, I became friends with Rick, who after high school and college went on to Harvard Law and became a powerful East Coast, Manhattan attorney. His girlfriend Sherri was sweet, kind, beautiful, and a brainiac. As the typical adolescent male, with hormones surging in the bloodstream, Rick couldn't stay away from this beauty Sherri. If I hung out with Rick, sooner or later, we would be over at Sherri's. My relief was Bernard, Sherri's father. It was he who helped draw me further into the wonders that medicine had to offer. Even though Bernard was not a physician, he was the chairman of the board of a local hospital that was also the hospital where I was born. Being involved in hospital life was one of Bernard's passions, and as a result of my close association with him, it became one of mine.

Many weekends when we visited Sherri, Bernard would invite me into his home office for a chat. Now the visits became much more interesting; ogling over Sherri wasn't as satisfying for me as it was for Rick. In fact, after a while, I would be disappointed if I didn't get a chance to visit with him.

Bernard was an extraordinarily intelligent and charismatic man. At five-foot-ten, with wavy, jet-black hair, he could have easily been mistaken for a younger Al Pacino. Bernard was in excellent shape and a very successful businessman. His mahogany office walls were covered with platinum awards, as well as pictures of him sailing his yacht in the Bahamas or on the lake, of skiing and playing tennis and golf with his buddies.

Bernard's business and hospital administrative achievements were only secondary to his modesty. I wouldn't say he had no ego, but it was very different than the ego and insecurity I have experienced from others. If he believed in something worthwhile, he would attack it with voraciousness matched by absolute integrity. He confidently believed he could make anything happen. But his focus was not on himself. His main hobby was medicine. As successful as he was as a businessman and in his outside interests, he was even more so as the CEO and president of the local hospital. I was in awe, and he was my mentor.

Many times Bernard and I would talk in his office about medicine—past, present, and future—for hours. He was enamored with those who went into medicine and referred to them as the "best and the brightest." His strongest values were integrity, dedication, and philanthropy. We talked about the dedication it took to be involved in the process of healing the sick and how the "art of medicine" was changing and evolving. If he knew a physician on staff wasn't coming from a place of absolute integrity, one who was greedy or had personal principles that weren't in line with appropriate patient care, he made a point of removing him from the hospital staff.

In later years, he would pick my brain about what was going on in the world of Obamacare. His daughter (and my friend) Sherri went on to become a renowned oncologist and researcher for Amgen. Sadly, she became stricken with multiple sclerosis, which resulted in her early demise. Even when she was faltering, she courageously continued to work, even helping to find a cure for my father's lymphoma. She was a true model of compassionate care.

Bernard was never quite the same after Sherri's death. His deep feelings regarding the loss of his daughter were only consoled by the love and compassion he had for his wife Barbara, daughter Kim, son Bruce, and the rest of his loving family. This wonderful man, who became a shell of his former self after multiple strokes, a ruptured colon, and nearly complete blindness, never let go of his passion for medicine and patients until the time of his passing. His example could not have been more inspiring, especially for a young, naïve teenager like myself who had a passion to help and heal. His passion for unconditional patient care became mine, and it was instrumental in motivating me to become a medical practitioner. Our talks helped to shape my thoughts about what I believe is important for healthcare today. He was my voice of reason many times in the midst of insanity, and I miss him dearly, with all my heart.

3. THE DREAM

*I have no idea what's awaiting me, or what will
happen when this all ends. For the moment I know
this: there are sick people and they need curing.*

Albert Camus

Before my dream of becoming a doctor could become a
reality, I knew I would need to achieve many things. I still
remember how proud my mother was of me when I was
elected to the National Honor Society in my junior year of
high school. She too had achieved this goal, and it pleased
her. She was also the valedictorian of her high school class, a
smart woman indeed. I still memorize the way she taught me,
focusing all my energy on the topic so it could be absorbed
as a permanent fixture in my brain, while repeating it over
and over again silently. One of her favorite sayings was that
you can achieve anything you want if you try hard enough. I
believe in her learning philosophy to this day. You need staying
power and dedication to accomplish anything; in fact, with

this mindset, no task is unachievable. I trusted her words and followed the path set before me. But my road to becoming a physician would be more arduous than I dreamed.

College decisions took me to a new crossroads. I didn't get into the local, six-year medical school program because even though I was in the local Kansas City metro area, I was still considered out of state. The state line runs through the middle of Kansas City, and I lived on the Kansas side of the state line, while the medical program was on the Missouri side. Now I had to choose between going to the state university or to an expensive private university. Ultimately, I chose the state university, so as not to be distracted by the fun and expense of the private university. The private university was also farther away, and although distancing myself from my family dynamics probably would have been an excellent choice for me, I still felt a responsibility to stay nearby. In some strange way, that sense of being needed helped to fill a void inside of me. I think I desperately needed to be in some kind of caring relationship to make up for what I was lacking emotionally. So off I went to the local university, to live in an apartment without distractions and make great grades so as to continue on my path to become a healer—while still remaining within earshot to help my family.

The pre-med grind was intense. The goal was excellent grades, especially in the pre-medical sciences. Every B pulled down your grade point average and cast doubt upon one's chance to be accepted to medical school. I can remember feeling exhausted after hours of memorizing organic chemistry equations, all the while wondering why it was necessary. (Actually, I still wonder why.) Nevertheless, it was required for acceptance to medical school, and everyone had to perform. The competition for A's was ever present. I had a friend who went to a private, southern school for college and had big problems getting into medical school. His school had a quota of how many A's professors gave out per class. In his class of two hundred organic chemistry students, only ten A's were granted. As a result, some students with averages over 90 percent received B's, further hindering their chances for getting into medical school. After a couple of years of this kind of competition, he transferred to a state university to help improve his odds for medical school acceptance. He was worn out and, he thought, defeated. Fortunately, he stuck with it, went to graduate school, did research, and got accepted to our local osteopathic medical school.

For many years after college, I would occasionally wake up in a cold sweat, anxious and distressed from a recurring nightmare. I would dream I had overslept and missed the final exam, jeopardizing my grades, graduation, and the chance to get into medical school. I've been a physician for over three decades, and I still sometimes wake up with this insane, disturbing dream. But I always feel relief upon waking up, realizing it was only a dream and I have transcended that time, now a live, well, and practicing physician.

After years of hard work, I was finally ready to apply to medical school. I had succeeded academically with a high grade point average and was ready to embark on the journey ahead. I had also done clinical research during the summers in a physiology lab and had co-published papers with a professor at the state medical school. After hours of tabulating data about the effects of nicotine on cat gut, which I had to dissect myself, while itching and sneezing throughout the duration because I was allergic to cats, I was ready to move on. My dedication and goals were steadfast. I took my medical college admission test, the MCAT, believing that nothing could stand in my way. I had been assured that with my pre-med course work, the MCAT would be a breeze. I didn't factor in my tendency to be a slow, methodical, test taker. Usually, I'm the last one to turn in an exam, and I found myself struggling to finish each section of the MCAT, sometimes not finishing the section at all. The distressing experience was further amplified by my scores, which were in the 45th percentile. Despite my superb grades, clinical research, and excellent letters of recommendation, my low MCAT scores took me out of the running and landed me on the alternate list. I still wanted to devote my life to others and use the compassion I had within me to succeed at becoming a physician, yet here I was at a major roadblock.

For the first time since I was drawn to medicine as a sixth-grade student, I had doubts about attaining my goal. Anger and frustration welled up inside of me, along with a feeling of helplessness. How could this happen to me after all of my hard work? Hadn't I proved myself worthy? Should my ability and aptitude to heal others really depend on a timed examination? When my sense of overwhelming despair and disappointment had cleared, I was left with an ache in my gut and the need to regroup. The final acceptance offers had been sent out. I didn't get into medical school from the alternate list, and now I would have to wait another year to try again.

I enrolled in some post-graduate courses, took a MCAT review course, and went back to working in my father's chemical plant. I soon realized more than ever that mixing and formulating chemicals was not my dream. Again, I was overwhelmed with the desire to get into medical school. Many times I felt like a ship off course and lost at sea.

I was not ready to give up on my dreams. I realized two things. First, I could never underestimate anything again. I learned that when you let your guard down, that's when the floor suddenly drops out from underneath you. Second, my goal to become a physician was not going to happen unless I figured out how to master the MCAT. I never forgot my mother's words, as the intelligent woman that she was when her mind wasn't altered with alcohol, that you could accomplish anything if you tried hard enough. In the mid-1970s, there was only one preparatory course for the MCAT: the Kaplan course. Obviously, this was long before the Internet, so I had to attend all courses in person. I immediately signed up for the course in St. Louis, Missouri, which was the nearest city. For the eight weekends prior to the test, I drove the five hours from Kansas City to St. Louis, checked into a motel, did coursework for eight hours a day on Saturday and Sunday, and then drove home. I took practice test after practice test, focusing on speed, and finally I felt ready. I took the MCAT and breezed through it, scoring in the 85th percentile. Soon afterward, I reapplied to medical school and was accepted without hesitation. Of course, my mother's philosophy proved correct: one can accomplish anything if he stays determined and tries hard enough.

Relieved but quite disgusted with this process, I was on a mission to prove my qualifications, even more than ever. Most medical students on the eve of starting their training are filled with excitement and enthusiasm for this new life and the challenges ahead. I, on the other hand, had a chip on my shoulder. My struggle to attain entry into medical school had changed me. Like a boxer waiting for a blindside punch, I had a focused, quiet intensity within that would not allow me to drop my guard for an instant. I think having the floor drop out from under me when I thought I had it all together was one of my greatest lessons. I will never forget it as long as I live. To this day, I never underestimate anything. Additionally, I am filled with gratitude and compassion. This roadblock helped me get to a place of positive energy, let go of the outcome in any situation, and accept that things happen exactly the way they should—and I continue to hold this philosophy today. I believe we get challenged and hit roadblocks exactly when we need to. These tests help us become more than we could ever be. Embracing roadblocks in a positive way gives you the opportunity to build your character and change anything that gets in the way of achieving your goals.

If you are a physician, I hope my stories help jog your own memories of how much dedication and focus it took to achieve your dreams. If you are patient, I hope you enjoy this ringside seat to the journey to and through medical school and appreciate the sacrifices physicians make on your behalf. Medical school and the training afterward are rigorous. But think of the possibilities if we, during our training, could also learn about the specialists who keep our mind and spirit healthy, to better integrate their care into our own protocol. We would not only have healthier patients, but healthier physicians as well.

4. THE GRIND

*Educating the mind without educating the heart is
no education at all.*

Aristotle

In the first two years of medical school, young doctors-to-be are learning the basics through study rather than practice. Occasionally, you may get a little clinical interaction, but basically those two years are about memorizing the human anatomy, cellular metabolism and structure, the physiology of the cardiovascular and nervous system, and the way drugs affect the human system. A grind like no other, it culminates in pathology, the study of disease on organ systems. If I had a dollar for every hour I spent studying, I'd be a rich man indeed.

These first years are grueling, taking a toll on one's time, mind, and body. It takes maximum concentration and focus to memorize the intricacies of the human body and condition.

All that studying culminated in tests, and those tests never end—even after a lifetime in the profession. Medical school requires an endless number of tests, as well as two parts of the national board testing. Afterwards, you must take tests to certify you in your specialty and subspecialty. Finally, even after you're certified, every ten years or so you have to take a recertification test.

Studying was easier for some students and harder for others. I was always going over something. I had to review a fact or concept at least three to four times before I was somewhat sure I retained it. On the other hand, one of my roommates, Dave, could barricade himself in a room for eight to ten hours straight without distraction and, after one thorough review, retain the information. His brain capacity was truly amazing. On the other hand, I was distracted easily and had to take frequent breaks. I could also, at my maximal limit of fatigue, put my head down on my desk, instantly fall into REM sleep, and wake up twenty minutes later refreshed, with a small puddle of drool on the table underneath my face.

Sometimes we barely had time to eat. One day, Dave suddenly broke from his concentrated learning with a voracious appetite; he went into the kitchen and began frying chicken. After he finished cooking and filled his plate with chicken, he immediately went back to the grind. A little later, I came out of my bedroom to take a break, and as I reached to turn on the light in the kitchen, I slipped on something, falling onto my ass and sliding all the way across the kitchen floor into the cabinets across from the door. The floor was so slippery, I had to pull myself up using the handles on the cabinet drawers, and when I turned on the light, to my dismay I saw grease and flour everywhere, as well as grease-spotted pieces of chicken sitting on paper towels all over the U-shaped kitchen counter. This was our life, barely having time to eat, cook, clean, or sleep in the middle of our concentrated efforts to learn everything we could on our quest to become physicians.

Those first two years of medical school were competitive and stressful for a number of reasons. A day or two after exams, we as students would anxiously wait for our scores to be posted. The anticipation was at times unnerving. Our grading system had three levels: superior, pass, and fail. If you failed a major section, it could set you back a year. Some of my classmates ultimately dropped out, were held back, or asked to leave when they couldn't perform or handle the pressure. This intensity was complicated by having little time to do anything else but study—and no money to-boot. I remember applying for low-interest student loans to help overcome the stress of being broke all the time. Taking out a loan was much better than receiving or borrowing money from my parents and being interrogated about what I was spending it on—although our spending involved little more than food, room, board, books, supplies, and tuition. It was hard not to feel like a horse traveling down a trail with blinders on. It took a decade to pay off my student loans after I started practicing medicine.

Serious romantic relationships during medical school were very difficult to keep. Unless you had a well-established and mature mate, most relationships didn't survive. For your relationship to succeed, your mate needed to embody the essence of support, care, unselfishness, and unconditional love. Most of us were too emotionally immature to engage in a relationship like that without messing it up. As a case in point,

I engaged in a somewhat intimate but short-lived relationship with another medical student in my class. Our relationship was based on convenience, mutual understanding of our situation, and our similar schedules, which eventually ended as our lives changed throughout our training. Sadly, most students who were married at the beginning of medical school were divorced when they finished. The couples who made it were usually older students in mature relationships, like former ICU nurses who had been better at patient care than their doctors and had decided to become physicians. With our focus on facts, diagnosis, and achievement, and our concerns about competing for a great residency, not much time was left for anything else. The best I could do was to squeeze in some exercise to reduce my stress and burn out the fuzzies. Reflecting back on these early years, I'm still amazed at the impact medical school had on me physically and emotionally.

As I mentioned before, in medical school I was on a mission to prove myself after initially being rejected, relentlessly driven to make great grades and be at the top of my class. One needed to excel during the first two years of basic sciences and the next two years of clinics. At the beginning of my junior year, I realized the fruits of my labor when I was elected to the Alpha Omega Alpha Honor Medical Society, which honored the top 10 percent of the medical school class.

How driven I was, and how helpless and demoralized I had felt. The roadblock I had endured with my MCAT scores made me want to cram my success down the acceptance committee's throat. The whole process weighed heavily on my heart for a long time. If I had given up, though, I would have most definitely missed my calling. For better or worse, that experience fueled my drive and ultimately pushed me to graduate the top of my class. Even then, I was still just as driven, as competition for the best residency spots was fierce.

What is it that motivates one to push ahead, no matter what obstacles lie in their way? Why doesn't everyone have the same drive or determination? Is it the fear of failure that drives us into medicine and makes doctors different? Yet with all this focus on external achievement, the old expression that you can't judge a book by its cover was still true. I knew that great performance was not a true measure of one's inner self or the ability to take great care of patients.

The gratification of helping others in need is an experience like no other. It heals the soul and comes from the heart and certainly forms my primary motivation as a physician. However, I know it's not true for everyone. I've known many physicians whose motivation came from a place of greed and ego, rather than dedication, integrity, and compassion.

I learned early on in medical school that some physicians really shouldn't have chosen healing as their profession, such as intelligent folks with unsteady hands as surgeons or poor judgment as clinicians. Some of them hide out in university or VA hospital settings. Some realize too late that they were better at research. Others are driven so much by greed that they push the envelope on indications for performing procedures. Early in my private practice, I remember a physical medicine specialist who would give a patient twenty to twenty-five epidurals for low back discogenic pain day after day at two thousand dollars a pop and not give it a second thought. Those physicians are the ones who rightly anger patients and other doctors and load wood onto the legal fire of malpractice. We must rid ourselves of that sort of travesty in patient care. However, although a patient's injuries due to negligence deserve dire consequences, starting the legal cascade never serves anyone well. We'll talk more about that in chapter 17.

5. REAL PATIENTS

The best way to find yourself is to lose yourself in the service of others.

Mahatma Gandhi

Our two-year academic grind culminated in the first part of the national boards. With that test and adequate grades under our belts, we could move on to the clinics, where the fun and challenge of integrating all our knowledge would begin. Clinical medicine was what we had been waiting for. Now we were taking care of real people with lives, families, faith, feelings, and fears. Clinics gave us the exciting opportunity to combine intuition, compassion, and facts and develop a sixth sense to achieve healing. It required both emotional stability and technical skills working in concert. We had been taught a lot about how the body functions and about how disease processes take place, but not much about the human spirit and how sickness affects you emotionally. So we learned how to draw blood, take blood pressures, and listen to people's chests and hearts with our stethoscope. There were labs to be evaluated and diagnoses to be presented to our attending staff.

Our teachers were the resident staff and the attending physicians, who didn't do much to prepare us emotionally for the challenges ahead. Some staff were better teachers than others. The Socratic method of interrogation, or putting us on the spot to the point of embarrassment and pointing out the flaws in our core evaluation and decision making, was the norm. One had to be up to date on his patients, labs, diagnosis, and history, and also needed to have read about the patient's condition and treatment. Being called on during rounds would leave a pit in your stomach, and occasionally I would feel the urge to rush to the toilet when my gut got too agitated. The pressure was almost intolerable.

Some of our staff physicians were unusually cruel. I remember a time during an abdominal surgery, when a fellow student and I were assisting Dr. A, one of our "legend in his own mind" general surgeons. Bill, the other student, had not adequately taped his eyeglasses to his forehead. When he leaned over to hold the retractors while looking into an abdominal wound, his glasses slipped from the bridge of his nose and fell into the wound. The staff surgeon pulled Bill's glasses out, threw them against the wall, and irrigated the wound thoroughly. Next, he grabbed Bill by his gown, took him across the room to an empty IV pole, and proceeded to circumferentially tie him to the pole with tape, immobilizing him and instructing him not to move or speak. Those types of situations filled us with fear and made it hard for us to function from a loving and compassionate place.

That said, fear can definitely motivate you to learn, as well as to ask for help. The sheer fear of the Socratic exam makes you search for all the available information about a patient and his care to avoid embarrassment. I'm not sure that the motivation to provide the best treatment possible overpowered our need not to appear to be an idiot in those early years. The responsibility was not yet given to us, but the need to prove ourselves was.

Teamwork was an important concept, and asking for help was imperative. We followed the old expression of "see one, do one, teach one." Occasionally, one faced doing a procedure with nothing much more than book knowledge, which definitely brought us to a new level of anxiety. When I was on surgery call as a medical student on a general surgery rotation, I was teamed up with another female medical student, Mary, to cover in-house problems. Mary was intelligent, with beautiful blonde hair, and was one of the more attractive students. One night I got a call from the head nurse to see a post-surgical male patient who couldn't urinate after his surgery and was quite uncomfortable. He needed to be catheterized, and I was enlisted. The only problem was I had never seen a foley catheter or inserted one. This was a dilemma, indeed.

I knew I couldn't ask the nursing staff to help me catheterize this patient. At this time in our training, the nurses did not do invasive-type procedures like this. I knew Mary was also on call, so I contacted her to see if she could help me. Her response was, "No problem," and she told me that she had catheterized one patient in the past. I can't tell you how relieved I was, and I met her in the nurses' station close to the patient's room. I had already assessed the patient, and Mary gave me a quick tutorial.

Together we went into the room. The patient was distended and in pain, due to the fact that he could not urinate. I explained the procedure to the patient as if I were an experienced pro. I laid out the catheter and the prep, put on my rubber gloves, pulled back the bed sheets, reached out and grabbed his manhood, prepped him, and feebly tried to insert the catheter to no avail. As I fumbled at my attempt, Mary spoke up and said, "Let me do it," and moved me aside. She proceeded in the same fashion, but this time, as this beautiful blonde grabbed this uncomfortable male patient, his response was to get an erection. Needless to say, I'm not sure who was more embarrassed: us or the patient. Mary was able to get the catheter into his bladder, but as soon as she did, because it was was so distended, urine shot everywhere, spraying us and the patient. We were finally able to hook the catheter to the bag and immediately had to remove ourselves from the room, as we could barely restrain our laughter and embarrassment. Once we regained our composure, we returned to the patient and apologized for making such a mess. The patient, so happy to be relieved of that intense bladder pressure, kindly thanked us. Our first attempt at teamwork wasn't a total flop, but as time went on, we learned how to diminish our fear and anxiety and achieve successful care of patients.

At times we went thirty-six hours or more without sleep. I learned how to catch fifteen- to twenty-minute naps sometimes by simply leaning against the wall or back in a chair. Sleep deprivation, combined with the challenge of patient care made it tough to think clearly, much less handle being interrogated by our attendings. Balancing knowledge, fatigue, personal life, and patient dedication—all while remaining compassionate—was quite a challenge. Long after I completed my training, the medical students started unions for student rights, which restricted excessive work hours. Unfortunately, that threw the balance back the other way; now, many new, young physicians start practice without a firm dedication to work ethics. Doctor's leaving in the middle of the patient care event at the end of their shift, regardless of resolution, doesn't work to the patient's best advantage unless it's done with a conscientious and compassionate transfer of care. I'll say more about this in chapter 7.

I can't emphasize the importance of intuition and compassion in caring for patients. That is truly the heart of healthcare. In medical school, so much time was spent on memorization and intellectual training and too little was spent on the emotional component. Many times physical illness and symptoms are emotional and can't be cured with a knife, plate and screws, or medicine. We all need to understand spiritual healing, which is based on heart, compassion, trust, reassurance, and presence. This type of healing helps a patient overcome illnesses that are not cured or affected by regular, Western medical treatment. This kind of spiritual healing can be an adjunct to Western medicine or used in place of it, and it usually involves using positive energy. Many times this is what our patients really need and want. Lesson number one is to be a good listener. A surgeon, for example, may quickly realize no procedure will help to cure a particular patient and his problem. His recognition of this reality and his openness and dedication to get the patient to the best healer for help is important if his skills are inadequate.

Some of my patients have asked me about alternative treatments that incorporate spiritual and emotional components of healing, and if they are not harmful, I readily endorse them. Understanding the emotional and spiritual needs of patients and integrating other alternative healers and their expertise into our medical knowledge is the essence of compassionate care. I realize this now more than ever, and I wish it had been taught in my early training. This kind of integrated, compassionate care is what we as practitioners should strive for and what patients should expect and seek out. We'll talk more about this in chapter 13.

6. EGO AND COMPASSION IN THE OPERATING ROOM

Too often we underestimate the power of a touch, a smile, a kind word, a listening ear, an honest compliment, or the smallest act of caring—all of which have the potential to turn a life around.

Leo Buscaglia

My wife always says that sometimes you can learn more by someone's bad example than by his good one, and I certainly learned a lot from dealing with others' egos in my training. Big egos can affect patient care negatively. My best example of this occurred when I was an early fourth-year medical student. I thought that I might want to be a heart surgeon, so I took a cardiothoracic surgery elective. I was on the rotation with Dr. B, who was chief of cardiothoracic surgery, otherwise known as Dr. Jekyll/Mr. Hyde. Outside the operating room, he was nice, diplomatic, and a strong clinician. Inside the operating room, he was a raving, abusive maniac with at least reasonable technical skills. He treated most operating personnel, students, and resident staff with intense anger and abuse, creating oppressive pressure in the operating room.

I was his primary surgical assistant, helping him with two open heart surgeries a day. A fifth-year resident took off for a fellowship after the first few days of my rotation, which left a team consisting of an intern, me, and a third-year student. For some reason, Dr. B disliked the intern. He would harvest the vein for the bypass surgery from the leg and then let me sew up the leg while he cracked the chest and went on bypass with the intern helping him. About the time I finished sewing up the leg and they finished going on bypass, he would dismiss the intern, asking him to go out on the floor, and then would have me be his sole surgical assistant. I was terrified. At first, I was elated to be able to close wounds and assist. Soon, though, the pressure became overwhelming, especially with the pressure that Dr. B put on all of us. By the end of the month, everything was a blur. I had a short vacation at the end of the rotation and went on a cruise with my parents and brother for a week. To this day, I still remember nothing of that trip.

That experience rid me of my thoughts of being a cardiothoracic surgeon. Maybe I would have felt differently if I had worked with a different attending surgeon. What I did learn was that if you antagonize those around you, it makes things worse. Calling your assistants sub-human primates, which Dr. B did, never helped. The more intensity placed on assistants, the worse everyone functions, and ultimately the patient's care will suffer. That type of negative energy definitely affects the functionality of the surgical team. So, early in my training, I learned a valuable lesson about stress and how to treat others.

I also learned something about the incredible power of compassion on my rotation with Dr. B. During one particular heart surgery, I was faced with an unforgettable life and death situation. I was assisting Dr. B on a bypass surgery when our patient, as we were getting ready to close the chest, went into cardiac arrest. The chest was nearly closed when it happened, and Dr. B had just scrubbed out and was in the scrub room just outside our operating room. When he was notified, he walked back into the operating room in a dramatic fashion, and without donning gloves or gown, he went back to the patient to reopen the chest, pulling out the stitches and cutting the sternal wires, and had me give open heart massage. Then he scrubbed back in and shocked the heart multiple times with small, operative shock paddles to try to resume a heartbeat. Nothing worked, and after five to ten minutes of this, he looked at me, his inexperienced fourth-year medical student, and told me to scrub out and tell the family that the patient wasn't going to make it.

The patient was the mayor of a small, local town and his two sons were deans of different departments at the University of Kansas, my alma mater and also the medical school I was attending. Knowing the patient and his family were influential, well-educated people didn't make the task at hand any easier.

I scrubbed out and began walking down a dimly lit corridor toward the waiting room in my sweat-soaked scrub top. I was literally trembling, my own heart just about coming out of my chest, as I thought about my grave responsibility. I emerged from this dark hallway into the brightly lit waiting room to tell this wonderful family the bad news. As I told them what was happening, their faces drained of color, and they went into a state of shock and disbelief, which resulted in the wife, sons, and myself breaking down into tears. It was one of the more overwhelming moments of my life. I felt totally helpless, and after regaining some composure, I reentered the operating room.

As I walked in, Dr. B was scrubbing out; the patient's condition had not changed. Dr. B had placed the patient on something called a balloon pump to help augment blood pressure, but all attempts were failing. He told me the patient wasn't going to make it and to scrub back in and close the chest. Dr. B left the room and sat down on a stool outside the operating room in the scrub area, his head in his hands in defeat.

As I was preparing to close the chest, even though my hands were shaking, I grabbed the wire for the sternum. Before I started to re-wire the sternum, the anesthesiologist looked at me and said, "Dr. B is in the scrub area. Why not shock the heart one more time?" I figured, *What did we have to lose?* I shocked the heart one more time with the intraoperative paddles. Miraculously, the heart started beating again. The anesthesiologist and I spent one full minute looking at the monitor, watching the heartbeat, and it was the longest minute of my life. When we finally got over our disbelief, I went out to the scrub area and asked Dr. B to please come back into the room. He was in shock as he also watched the monitor, and then he said, "Oh, no. It's just the balloon pump. Turn it off." We did, yet the heart continued to beat. He quickly scrubbed back in, and once he reentered the room again, he instructed me this time to tell the family that the patient might live. I had already been faced with sharing the news of this poor man's probable untimely death, and now I was charged with breaking this news to the family. Again, I walked down that dimly lit corridor into the bright waiting room. When the family saw me come through the door, they rushed to me for any news, and this time I was able to give them some hope for survival. The family embraced me tearfully, and together we experienced this rollercoaster of emotions: compassion, sadness, hope, anger, frustration, and the fear of facing the unknown.

That difficult month with Dr. B gave me one of the greatest gifts in my training. I learned about compassion, the importance of never giving up, the power of positive energy, and the disruption of negative energy. Those lessons helped shape my own approach with patients in difficult or stressful situations to this day. So much about patient care has to do with coupling knowledge with and approaching patients from a place of compassionate care, love, and positive energy. This approach positively affects the ultimate result, which should be the best possible healing for our patients. The joy that comes from hitting one's mark when caring for a patient is still secondary to the patient's healing itself. Dr. B's patient ultimately survived after being in a mental fog for some time, and he finally regained full mental and physical capacity.

When I graduated from medical school, we had our own private graduation ceremony, and we were also included in the University of Kansas commencement ceremony for the entire university. That ceremony included walking downhill into the football stadium. Along the way to the stadium, the path was lined with professors in their caps, gowns, and doctoral sashes. They greeted graduates, smiling and congratulating them. Halfway to the stadium, I received one of the most memorable honors of my life. Just ahead of me, I saw two different deans on opposite sides of the path break out of the greeting line and approach me. With handshakes and hugs, the two sons of the mayor congratulated me and thanked me for what I did to console them and to help save their father's life. To write about it even now brings tears to my eyes and fills me with loving compassion. I will never forget that moment, and many other moments like that, for as long as I live. We can achieve so much simply by being positive, loving, and full of integrity.

At the end of medical school, after being exposed to multiple aspects of the field of medicine, we had to make a career choice, based on what we were best capable of and compatible with. At first I thought I wanted to be a cardiologist, and then a cardiothoracic surgeon, but after my experience with Dr. B, it didn't seem like the right fit. I had taken many surgical electives, and I decided, for many reasons, that I was best suited to be an orthopedic surgeon.

In the field of orthopedics, I found with someone's injury, fracture, or other physical condition, I could quickly respond with an effective intervention that would soon get him or her back to their normal lives, as restoring near-normal skeletal and ligamentous anatomy usually took less than three to six months. Helping someone in pain or who was disabled was extremely gratifying. I usually didn't have to chase after chronic illness, and I was able to help take care of patients after they underwent surgical treatment. The rehabilitation after someone's injury or surgery was many times grueling, and it took as much on-going focus as it did surgical skills to help guide the patient to healing both physically and emotionally.

Learning how to respond to different people's personalities and their response to pain or injury has been fascinating. I realized that to do my job well, I needed skills in technical surgery, medical and pain management, psychology, physical and occupational therapy, compassion, and an energy that brought it all together. I have now also realized that to do my job to the fullest, I need to understand how spirituality and Eastern medicine influence healing. I have come to incorporate some of those approaches into my care and now realize that a combination of all these approaches helps to achieve optimal healing.

When I finished my training in medical school, I was accepted to an orthopedic internship and residency. I embraced it with all of my energy, but I still felt a void in my personal and social life. I felt the need to have some semblance of a family that wasn't dysfunctional and someone I could share my life with. It wasn't enough for me to just take care of patients; I felt like I needed a personal connection on a deeper level.

I ended up reconnecting with a girlfriend from college in those early residency years. Of course, the reasons the relationship didn't work to begin with years before hadn't disappeared, but I ignored them for the time being, figuring they could be worked out. Of course I could work it all out. I was the physician, and I was also the caretaker. It took me almost two decades of a failing marriage to realize that I really could not repair someone else's issues or problems, as a physician or a caretaker, but I did learn a very valuable lesson about what would work and what wouldn't work in a deep, interpersonal relationship with another person. I wish I would have had the emotional maturity sooner to realize the balance was not right for me. We experienced many years of infertility and sadness as well, but in later years, I was blessed with three beautiful children. I finally had to separate from that relationship because it was not good for my soul, which was in pain and filled with conflict. I did not want my children to grow up thinking an unhealthy relationship was the norm.

A couple of years later, I met a woman with the same first name as my last, the greatest woman I could have ever dreamed of, and my life was transformed as a result. With Rose, I found the balance in life I had been missing, a balance that comes from connecting with another person on a deep, interpersonal level and experiencing unconditional love. This balance is enhanced by two emotionally mature people cheering each other on to be their best selves through effective communication and respect for each other's needs and desires and by inspiring each other to follow their dreams. I was blessed to find her, and we married and blended her two fine sons with my children when they were young. Even though we spent years dealing with two emotionally immature ex-spouses who tried to dismantle our relationship with our children and our marriage, Rose was a dedicated parent to all our children, as was I, and luckily the end result was five incredible young adults. We are honored to share our lives with these wonderful children.

7. THE NEW PHYSICIAN GRADUATES

I think modern medicine has become like a prophet offering a life free of pain. It is nonsense. The only thing I know that truly heals people is unconditional love.

Elisabeth Kubler-Ross

As a physician practicing for over thirty years, I'm more satisfied now than I've ever been. It took me a long time to find a practice setting where I felt at home and free to practice without restriction, approaching patients with an open heart, but I believe I've now found it at Palo Alto Foundation Medical Group. My colleagues are all top notch; many are not only on the cutting edge of medicine, but also my friends. I love to learn new techniques from my colleagues so I can practice medicine at a higher level of excellence. When you look forward to going to work each day, that energy gets transmitted through your care. I believe this environment is mandatory for success.

Also, I don't see what I do as work. I was led here, and for me, medicine is more like a vocation. Dedicated professionals, caring for others with compassion and without ego or a desire for personal gain, will bring about healing. Patients should look for this kind of healing environment—and so should physicians.

In fact, viewing your job as a vocation may be the only way to bring about the dedication required. Physicians spend a lot of time in the trenches caring for our patients, and it's demanding. During and after training, I did whatever it took to get the job done, even if I had to sacrifice my free time. I can remember one time when at twelve thirty in the morning I got a call from a friend whose eleven-year-old daughter smashed her finger in a door at a slumber party. He called me on my cell phone to ask me what to do. The young associate on call at the emergency room had suggested sending her to the university hospital for care, and her dad was beside himself. So at one in the morning, I came in, calmed my friend's daughter, and repaired her finger in the emergency room. The father and daughter were so thankful and relieved that for years afterwards, whenever I saw her she would proudly hold out her hand and show me her finger. That "old school," patient-first philosophy is always gratifying for both the physician and the patient, and it is the right thing to do.

I can't tell you how many times my life has been interrupted by my chosen profession. I can't even remember how many parties, games, movies, and family events I had to leave or couldn't attend due to my commitment to being a dedicated physician. Family time is certainly sacred to me. What's even more sacred is having a spouse and family who understand when emergencies come up that are out of your control and who cheer you on to "take care of business." Many times I would come home from work after a busy day, and not long after, the doorbell would ring. Some neighbor or friend would be at my door with an injury. Earlier he had talked to Rose, my amazing bride, who had directed him to our home, regardless of how it might impact our night or weekend. Support like that makes for an incredible home life.

However, balance is important as well. At one point in my career, I spent a decade taking care of trauma patients at a trauma center, spending countless hours away from home treating complicated issues far beyond my comfort level. My work situation was so out of balance for my family and myself that I had to leave that practice setting, which allowed me the opportunity to find and enjoy my present job. Dedication and balance between work, spouse, family, friends, and outside interests are imperative to a successful practice and a happy life.

When I was in training, no unions or movements set standard hours for medical students or residents. You didn't clock in or clock out when someone was sick or simply leave when your eight-hour shift was up. As a parent, if your child is sick with a high fever and you have to be up all night nursing him back to health, that's what you do. Physicians should be the same way. Yes, balance is important, and without it your life can be left in shambles. But I fear some of the new generation of physicians have lost some of the dedication and compassion engrained in our "old school" training. The belief that we treat everyone as family or friend needs to be reinserted back into medicine. That's our future. For friends and family, we always go the extra mile out of compassion. We shouldn't resist taking on a job because it conflicts with our exercise spin class schedule or delay a child's early morning operation until the afternoon because the physician wants to sleep in. Trying to keep a child NBO (nothing by mouth) all day is miserable for the child and his parents. We need to practice medicine in accordance with what's in the best interest of our patients, regardless of our own needs.

I strongly believe medical training should require compassion training that encourages a physician to step into the shoes of his patients. Physicians like Dr. Rachel Remen have been instrumental in teaching compassion to medical students and physicians early in their training, and I believe courses like hers should be mandatory in all medical schools today.

Young physicians and their patients should also be focused on developing a new systematic approach to medicine, which should include insurance and tort reform as well as pharmaceutical revamping, as we'll talk more about in part 3. The entire system needs to change. As physicians, we're seeing too many patients, experiencing a shortage of doctors, and watching reimbursements going down. Why would anyone want to go into medicine if the reimbursement was so poor that it didn't match his time, effort, and energy?

The costs of becoming a physician are beginning to outweigh the benefits. Not only has college and medical education tuition skyrocketed, leaving many with hundreds of thousands of dollars in debt before they can generate a productive income, but the thought of politicians, insurance agents, and attorneys dictating how you can practice medicine makes the profession feel like an uphill battle. Excellent physicians are leaving medicine or retiring early, and I don't want patients to miss out on healing or physicians to feel pushed out of their calling.

But if physicians, healthcare professionals, and patients work together, I have hope we can come up with solutions that result in a renaissance of compassionate care that benefits all parties—as we'll explore in the remaining sections.

PART TWO

Healing the
Physician / Patient Relationship

*I think we learn from medicine everywhere that it
is, at its heart, a human endeavor, requiring good
science but also a limitless curiosity and interest in
your fellow human being, and that the physician/
patient relationship is key; all else follows from it.*

Abraham Verghese

8. THE PRACTICE OF MEDICINE

The aim of medicine is to prevent disease and prolong life, the ideal of medicine is to eliminate the need of a physician.

William J. Mayo

After I completed my training, my first practice setting was a very small, private practice with two associates who were limited emotionally as well as technically. One was intelligent and technically adequate, but he had poor communication skills and, therefore, poor outcomes. The other associate had the worst combination of all: he was intelligent, had a huge ego, communicated poorly, and was a terrible technician. He didn't ask for help and had multiple liability suits pending. Overall, their results were generally poor, and the whole experience was a bust.

In many ways, much like my experience with Dr. B, I learned quite a lot about how *not* to practice medicine, and for that, I'm grateful. Surprisingly, from the outside, that practice looked competent and inviting, but not from the inside. It was a painful experience for me, as a thinking, feeling human being, to go through that training, so needless to say, I couldn't wait to leave. I only lasted a little over a year.

My next practice experience was as an employee and then, two years later, a partner at a great multi-specialty group in San Diego, California. The group had about one hundred physicians when I first arrived, and six years later, it had grown to over three hundred physicians. The group was excellent and well run, with wonderful teamwork and camaraderie. I still would be there if I hadn't returned to the Midwest to take on a new challenge, helping to build an orthopedic program at a private hospital and attending to two parents with cancer.

In Kansas City, I began as a hospital employee, which evolved into a corporate/HMO employee, and then finally I was a private practitioner in a larger orthopedic group. I witnessed the progression of corporate buyouts, and I saw how a large national corporation could completely turn around a wonderfully satisfying private hospital. For me, it was hard to watch the personality and character of this hospital change and take on a corporate structure. The care was still good, but it was just different. Returning to the private practice model wasn't much easier, though. The rising malpractice premiums and the fight within the insurance carriers were miserable. Again, more learning experiences.

During part of my orthopedic practice in the Midwest, I found myself doing a lot of inner city trauma, which was arduous and unfortunately did not provide much personal satisfaction. Finally, with the help and support of my wife, I got the courage to design my life. I began to look for an opportunity that offered what I thought was the epitome of how medicine should be practiced. With open eyes, lo and behold, I found an incredible multi-specialty group in the San Francisco Bay Area. I believe this group embodies how medicine will be practiced in the future, and I have happily remained there to this day.

Although one's definition of the ideal practice setting is definitely personal, in my opinion, my present setting would be hard to beat. In our large medical group, we have a wonderful electronic medical record (EMR) system that allows all of us to know what kind of care we are providing to patients and to collaborate together. Luckily, EMR systems are becoming the norm and should be the norm for the future. We can pull up radiographs, labs, tests, and other pertinent evaluations online in the office and review them from home as necessary.

We can easily connect with our staff and ask unanswered questions online with our colleagues and our patients. The information exchange is utterly amazing. In a group setting like this, I can walk up the stairs or to an adjacent building and take a look at a patient for a colleague and assist in his care immediately. Education, competence, prevention, communication, and excellence in caring is our mission. Our physicians are all handpicked with scrutiny to make sure that the physician and the group match perfectly.

Our group is big enough to be self-insured for liability, and we have a team of businessmen who negotiate our contracts. Physician turnover is minimal, and doctor and patient satisfaction are maximal. When you can approach an illness or surgery while collaborating with confident, compassionate, and caring colleagues, the resulting positive energy creates the ultimate healing outcome. The patient and doctors are both happy. What more could one ask for?

9. AVOID THE TERRIBLE TRIAD: EGO, GREED, AND FEAR

When we practice loving kindness and compassion, we are the first ones to profit.

Rumi

The purpose of human life is to serve, and to show compassion and the will to help others.

Albert Schweitzer

I'd like to take a moment to talk directly to patients now. As we've seen, physicians go through an arduous course to get to where they can start taking care of patients. It includes not only medical school and training, but it also includes their past, their upbringing, their true nature, and their soul as a healer. So what makes physicians good? What should a patient look for in a physician? These are important questions for you to ask if you want to get the care you need to heal your illness or ailment.

Physicians who are practicing medicine are all relatively intelligent folks; otherwise, they would never have gotten to the level that they did to achieve their MD or DO status.

As a board-certified physician, I always recommend that my patients seek out those certified in their respective fields for their care. In the 1930s, the American Board of Medical Specialties was established to set standards for physicians, and one becomes certified when he meets these standards. Board certification has advanced the expertise that physicians share with their patients today and has worked well. Peer-defined standards are imperative for all healing practitioners. There is no place in healing for inadequacies.

But even if you have found an intelligent, board-certified physician, certain characteristics can alter the way he practices medicine and, unfortunately, can adversely affect patient care. They include what I call the terrible triad: ego, greed, and fear.

EGO

What exactly do I mean by ego? It's very simple. If a physician doesn't get help from other colleagues or refuses to entertain other viewpoints because he or she thinks they know more than anyone else, that's ego. The best description of ego that I've heard is from Dr. Deepak Chopra. He describes ego as "edging God out." Working from a place of strong ego limits our judgment and affects patient care adversely.

As physicians, we can never know enough. I'm not talking about simple and straightforward treatment plans for clear-cut illness; I'm talking about complicated situations that are difficult to diagnose or treat. In cases like these, a compassionate healer considers all options for treatment and leaves no stone unturned.

Unfortunately, as I have previously stated, I have worked

with practitioners who were so full of themselves that they refused to believe that the care they provided was actually harmful. A surgeon who is a terrible technician, an internist who misses a diagnosis or generates an ineffective or harmful treatment plan, or an oncologist who isn't up to date on cutting-edge cancer treatment plans are a few examples of physicians who should either find a new career or a different specialty. A bad outcome usually results in an angry patient and/or family, sometimes followed by legal action.

That said, I believe that the "God complex" that used to characterize physicians is not as prevalent now as it was two or three decades ago. When I first started practicing, I remember many physicians who presented themselves as beyond reproach, no matter what they did or how things turned out with their care. Today, a plethora of excellent physicians to choose from and an abundance of hungry attorneys have limited the number of those physicians who stand at their altar and proclaim that their word, judgment, or treatment is second to none. Many patients now can get a second opinion about their care or can simply look on the Internet and research their physician or the latest treatments. Access to information has never been better, and you can get star ratings not only for movies and restaurants, but for physicians.

This abundance of information is good, but it is also potentially confusing for the patient. Too many choices can also hold someone back from making a good choice. Also, star ratings may not reveal the underlying personality flaws associated with strong ego. I've seen poor physician ratings that had very little to do with the physician; the patient was merely upset with his bill because he did not understand what was covered by his insurance. I've also seen poor ratings due to unrealistic patient expectations or a survey sample based on a very small number of patients surveyed. Online evaluations and ratings still leave a lot to be desired.

Ego can also prevent physicians from giving their optimal effort to find the best treatment for their patients. Optimally, a physician will fully research the presenting problem and, if appropriate, find the best specialist for the patient. This extra effort would result in an excellent treatment plan with optimal results, a patient who is no longer experiencing fear but peace and serenity, and a healing relationship based on trust. My family and friends have approached me many times for an opinion unrelated to my specialty. I enjoy researching things, especially if I can help someone receive the treatment he needs. I have plenty of friends in different specialties, and if I can somehow make a difference for someone, the effort is worth it to me. I'm sure many of my colleagues do the same thing.

GREED

Like ego, greed is found in every profession. My mentor Bernard's favorite quote was, "What does a greedy man want? Response: just a little bit more." When a person is motivated by greed, many times his judgment is clouded and the result will most certainly not benefit all. If a physician consistently orders unnecessary procedures, the reason is likely greed. When he suggests a questionable treatment and persuades a patient to comply, and the physician benefits, the reason is also likely greed. When he bills for more time with the patient than he has spent or procedures he hasn't done, then that is not only greed, but fraud.

Have I known physicians who have tried to manipulate the system for their own personal gain? Unfortunately, yes, I have. Fortunately, I am now part of a group that does not tolerate greed in any form. Let me give you a good example.

When I first started my present job at the large, multi-specialty group in the Bay Area, I was hired to help build the orthopedic expansion in one of their divisions. I packed up my home, my wife, and my family in Kansas, and we moved cross country to engage in this new endeavor. We were excited about this new opportunity, but I was also somewhat sad at leaving my patients and some of my family behind.

When I arrived, I discovered that about two months prior to my arrival, a community doctor had been hired to work with me. I also received a warning from another colleague that this new physician may have some patient-care issues and was overcharging to his benefit. As an experienced physician with tenure, I figured I could handle whatever came my way.

During the first week at my new practice, I was exposed to this physician in the office and in surgery. Within days, after working with this physician, I realized that even though he had a pleasant personality and had trained at a top university, he was quite inept as a surgeon and had questionable patient-care skills and judgment. I became very distraught, and for the first time, I wasn't really quite sure how to proceed. After moving my wife and children across the country to start a new life in a new place, I came home one night in despair and confided in my wife that there was no way I could work with this physician because of his ethics and the way he took care of patients. It was clear he was motivated by greed and not by patient care.

My intuitive wife wisely said, "I agree; you can't work there or work with him if that's the situation."

I spent a sleepless night contemplating how to proceed, and the next day I decided I needed to meet with the medical director of our division to discuss my thoughts. We set up a meeting, and when I sat down with her, I found myself quite anxious, with my heart pounding. I began to describe some of my observations of poor patient care during that week. I told her that I hadn't hired this man and that I was hopeful for a wonderful practice experience with this group, but if he stayed, I felt I would have to leave. I laid all my cards out on the table. I just couldn't tolerate working with someone who was not giving his best effort to take care of his patients.

To my relief, she replied that the medical group supported me completely, and they had heard some complaints too. I was asked to record examples of poor care and patient complaints, which I researched and provided. Within a week, he was gone. The medical director, who didn't really even know me other than my credentials, trusted me enough to support my position, based on my compassionate concern for patient care. My concerns were in alignment with her ethics and our group's mission. She remains a wonderful friend to this day, and she and the others in my group work together in the best interest of our patients.

When a physician focuses on money rather than care, he loses his credibility and hopefully his medical license. As for me, I try to ignore the reimbursement amount for procedures so my decisions are based on the patient's best interest. When I started my training, I was a purist; my ultimate goal was healing. That is still my goal. The money, fame, and status that can result from success in any profession can influence one's priorities. Making decisions to benefit the patient's healing, untainted by greed, is not only a matter of best outcomes, it's also a matter of integrity.

FEAR

What would a physician have to fear? Well, first off, he or she may fear that he isn't up to par with his peers. If he feels his knowledge or technical skills are not as good as others, fear may cause him to overcompensate in a variety of ways. He may beat his own drum about his accolades. He may refuse to study more, get extra training, or change specialties in response to poor performance. What then transpires is ineffective or even damaging treatment. This situation is the exception rather than the rule, but these exceptions are dangerous.

Of course, complications and poor results can happen with any medical or surgical intervention, even with the best treatment or care. The human being is complex, and medicine alone does not heal. Desire, intention, and belief all play a huge role. That's not what I'm talking about. I'm talking about physicians whose fear prevents them from following the ultimate goal to "do no harm."

I can remember how uncomfortable and fearful I was during one of my first solo cases as an orthopedic resident. I had scrubbed with my staff surgeon for a lumbar disc removal many, many times. On a routine surgery day, we were to do a lumbar disc excision on a patient, and my staff surgeon, Dr. J, told me to position, prep, and drape the patient. After I finished, Dr. J was not present, and I asked the OR staff to call him. He called back into the room and, over the speaker phone, instructed me to make the skin incision and expose the area of the spine we were working on. With trepidation, I began with the skin incision and slowly completed the exposure. After exposed, I had him paged again, and he called in and said, "Start removing the disc, and I'll be right there." I started to sweat, but slowly and cautiously, I began removing small pieces of the disc. Time passed and soon there was no more disc to be removed. My rapid heart rate returned to normal. Again, there was no Dr. J, and he was paged again. When he called in, I told him what I had done, and he told me to close the wound. As I was putting on the wound dressings, into the operating room walked Dr. J. He looked at the patient, told me everything looked great, and walked out. I had been through a myriad of emotions, including fear, anxiety, and—at the end—satisfaction and confidence. Dr. J had worked with me and knew I was ready to do the case solo—even though I didn't know it myself. I took on the challenge and responsibility and overcame the fear. I was left with a confidence to take on more challenges and a cautiousness to do no harm.

The insecure, fearful, and sometimes lazy physician tends to order excessive laboratory tests and x-rays and inappropriate consultations. A physician who is in fear of being sued for malpractice does the same thing. His concerns about being sued force him to overcompensate and many times drive up the costs of medical care, which we'll talk more about in chapter 16.

A positive, caring physician, one committed to his patient's best interest, will naturally team up with his colleagues and focus on the patient. A physician can ensure a successful doctor/patient relationship by starting off merely listening to his patient's ills and being compassionate. Most patients want to be heard and understood. We're all being trained to do simple things like maintain eye contact and not interrupt a patient for at least the first thirty to sixty seconds of a discussion to help achieve successful communication. Caring physicians who are truly interested in their patients, even if they can't achieve a cure with their best efforts, will still avert liability. A happy physician who talks to his patients about their problems, treatment, and needs will succeed, as will the patient. The more the physician can ease a patient's fears, while avoiding fear himself, the more the energy will flow in the right direction. Of course, adding technical and diagnostic skills and using a team of caregivers is even better. Lastly, physicians should not hesitate to refer patients with complicated issues to others with more expertise for optimal outcomes, just as patients need to ask for other opinions when the path toward healing isn't crystal clear.

10. FINDING BALANCE

I have faith in the unlimited, loving power of the universe.

Louise Hay

As a Libran, I always tend to focus on balance. How can we get back to a state of balance in healthcare? First and foremost, physicians need to get back to the basics of patient care. Today physicians often find themselves running an office, getting insurance reimbursements, negotiating contracts, and dealing with healthcare conglomerates—in addition to caring for patients, which is supposed to be their first priority.

Our multi-specialty group is part of a foundation that not only takes care of the business and contractual aspects of practicing medicine, but also negotiates and deals with the insurance companies as well. Insurance companies, hospital corporations, and HMO groups are often focused on the bottom line, their own corporate profit, so physicians do need to protect their interests. This arrangement allows us to do what we do best, which is take care of patients. I have known a number of busy physicians who have left the day-to-day office management up to their office manager, only later to find out that this employee has done a poor job or has even embezzled from their corporation. I would be naïve to pretend that profits for physicians in corporations aren't important. I also have to be honest about the fact that most physicians aren't very good businessmen. Physicians have to have extensive training to get started and have long, stressful workweeks. They are constantly in training, going to CME (continuing medical education) courses and workshops. Their job is arduous and intense. Some choose to teach part time, and others go out to underserved areas on medical missions. The role they chose as a physician many times takes them away from their spouse, family, and friends. Their life is hard to keep in balance, and when out of balance, many things like divorce, depression, common sickness, and even death can occur. All this brings me back to the question at hand: how do we achieve the best balance between our practice, our spouse and/or family, our social life, and even our personal health?

Right before I finished my orthopedic residency and started practice, I took an elective with two very fine hand surgeons in private practice. One was an orthopedic surgeon and another was a plastic surgeon, and they both had extensive microvascular skills. In the city I lived in at the time, they handled many of the re-implantation surgeries that were necessary when someone cut off a finger or part of his hand. When someone accidentally cuts off a finger, the tissue is viable for implantation for only a short time period. That meant nearly every patient who needed reimplantation was sent to them, and when that happened, they would have to stop everything they were doing, whether it involved their home life, patient care, or other surgeries, and run to the operating room to start the preparation and then continue with the surgical treatment. Many times these surgeries would last twenty to thirty hours. The work was long and tedious, and a lot of it was done under a microscope. It had a profound physical and emotional strain on everyone involved with the care.

I've never known two men to work harder. After they would finish these long surgical cases, they would quickly regroup and then spend the next two or three days seeing the patients they had cancelled and resuming the other surgeries that had been put on hold. Sometimes this would extend their days to eight or nine o'clock at night—often only to be followed by another injury that would throw them back into the same cycle.

When I finished that two-month rotation, I was definitely worn out, and I also realized that that wasn't my idea of a balanced practice. I have the ultimate respect for these two physicians, and sadly the intensive work took its toll. The next year, the orthopedic surgeon, who was in his early forties, had a heart attack in the airport on his way to a medical meeting and passed away in the airport. It was a huge loss to our community. Also during that year, the plastic surgeon, who was a bit older, got so run down that he collapsed one day after finishing an incredibly busy work week. He had contracted meningitis and encephalitis and was intubated in an ICU for six weeks. He did recover, but only to find that he had some residual neurologic damage and was partially paralyzed on one side. He could no longer effectively operate as a surgeon. He still continued to practice medicine, but not as a surgeon, which was another tragedy. Sadly, their balance was off, and unfortunately, they paid dearly.

In our search for balance, the practice of medicine continues to evolve. I think I have finally found the best model for balanced care that is a win-win for the physician, corporation, and most importantly, the patient. I believe it's a setting like the one I'm currently working in, where the medical group is multi-specialty and physician run and works hand in hand with a corporation or foundation that has the business experience to manage all the clinic and insurance contractual functions. As I mentioned previously, our group is self-insured to minimize legal and malpractice concerns, and we have our own internal risk management team to evaluate problems, complications, and patient concerns. We are able to provide electronic medical records; radiographic tests and ancillaries like MRI, CT, and PET scanning; oncology perfusion; sleep centers; and surgery centers, which allows better patient access to care. We have centers of excellence that combine the best of technology, physicians, and equipment to effect positive healing. We use variation reduction to look at what produces the best results. We are concerned about patient and physician satisfaction, and at the same time, we try to rein in excessive costs. We treat everyone—no matter what insurance he carries. Everyone is happy when costs are contained, profits are maximized, and patient care is outstanding for all, not just for the people who can afford it.

It takes a large group of dedicated professionals to combine resources, share ideas, and work as a team to help develop and design effective healthcare-delivery systems. Studying successful systems like ours (the Palo Alto Medical Foundation), the Mayo Clinic, Sharp Rees Stealy Medical Group, and the Cleveland Clinic would be a great first step toward preserving the future of healthcare in our country.

11. APPROACHING ALLIED HEALTH

*Our task must to be free ourselves by widening our
circle of compassion to embrace all living creatures
and the whole of nature and its beauty.*

Albert Einstein

Physicians must not forget that the best results do not
come from successful procedures alone—they often depend
on the people physicians engage to help them. They cannot
do their work alone! Success in surgery or medicine depends
on many levels of the healthcare system. I can't tell you how
thankful I am to have the best help from my other colleagues
and allied healthcare workers.

Let me give you an example of how all the tiers of care can
work together to achieve excellent results. My patient Milly
comes to see me with a sore knee. After I take a good history
and a thorough physical exam, I come up with some treatment
ideas. Milly has had a couple of previous arthroscopic surgeries,

she takes her arthritis medicine, and she has had cortisone and hyaluronic acid injections. Cortisone helps decrease the inflammation in the knee, and hyaluronic acid injections, like Synvisc, Supartz, and a host of other brands, increase the viscosity of the fluid inside the joint and help create an internal buffer. Many times those shots help anywhere from thirty days to six months or a year. Sometimes, they don't help at all. Now, at age sixty-five, Milly can hardly walk more than a block or two without pain. Her quality of life leaves something to be desired. She can't walk to exercise her heart and can't travel or chase her grandkids around. During our discussion, Milly decides that it's finally time to replace her knee.

Now I have to educate her about what she's in for. I tell her that when she's cleared medically by one of my colleagues, she will be following a protocol after surgery that usually involves many allied healthcare workers, such as nurses and physical and occupational therapists, to achieve the best result. My surgical skills are only part of the treatment; her motivation in working with the other health professionals is the rest. She agrees, and the next phase of treatment begins.

To prepare for surgery, Milly first visits with my nurse, who educates her about the process and orders the necessary preoperative labs, x-rays, an EKG, and a chest x-ray. She also sets up visits with her family practitioner, internist, cardiologist, and other appropriate consultants. My nurse also arranges for her to have a blood thinner after her surgery. (A blood thinner like Lovenox or Coumadin will help prevent post-operative blood clots.)

Next, Milly visits with my surgery scheduler, who sets up a surgical date, obtains insurance approval, and gives Milly an education notebook on joint replacement. Prior to surgery, Milly goes to the hospital, confers with the anesthesiologist, and attends a class at the Center for Joint Replacement. At that class, nurses and therapists talk with her about the surgery process and rehabilitation.

The day of surgery arrives, and after a pleasant admission process, the holding area nurses prep Milly, check her labs, insert IVs, start antibiotics, go over the consent form, and hopefully allay Milly's fears. Many times my joint replacement patients get a spinal epidural catheter placed to control post-operative pain and discomfort, which can decrease the need for a full general anesthetic. After seeing the anesthesiologist and myself, she is off to the operating room.

Prior to her arrival, the room has been prepared with the highest level of sterility by OR personnel and the nurse; the surgical tech had prepared the operating table with the instruments for the best possible procedure. An implant representative is usually present before and during the surgical procedure to ensure that the correct implants are available and also to assist with any decision making. In the room, after Milly has fallen asleep, her leg is prepped by a circulating nurse and draped by the surgeon and his assistant, usually a physician's assistant.

After the surgery, a recovery room nurse immediately attends to Milly to make sure she is stable. A lab technician comes in to do blood work, and an orthopedic technician comes in to put Milly's leg in a continuous passive motion machine. An x-ray technician comes in to take a picture of her knee. Once Milly is stable in her recovery room, she is moved to the floor.

On the floor, a floor nurse and nurse's aide settles Milly into her room. Over the next two or three days, the nursing staff and ancillary personnel closely monitor her pain, wounds, blood, urine, eating, and activity. Almost immediately a physical therapist starts working with her twice a day and an occupational therapist starts helping her with activities in daily living. A social worker meets with her and her family about her needs when she goes home or if she needs to temporarily go to a skilled nursing unit. This team of allied healthcare workers prepares Milly and her family for her return home.

When she is ready to leave, home visits are scheduled with a home physical therapist or nurse. Once home and ambulatory, Milly will then return to see me for frequent monitoring and to see outpatient physical therapy until she steps back into her new and improved life with a new knee.

This is only one small example of the multifaceted care a patient can receive; compared to a patient in a life or death situation, this process might seem simple. But the point is that if Milly's team of allied healthcare workers weren't involved to the extent that they were, the outcome and success of her treatment might indeed be very different. Without the team in place, our results are quite limited; with them in place, our successes are limitless. An orderly's cleaning of the operating room can make the difference between an uncomplicated outcome and a catastrophic post-operative infection. The head nurse and her team's organization of the operating room and set protocols can make the difference between a successful surgery and a surgery filled with delays, causing a less than optimal outcome. Surgical results do not need to be tested by a poorly prepared operating room lacking the right equipment or help. After surgery, a skilled physical therapist or occupational therapist can make the difference between a full recovery and lifelong struggle. Their compassion and caring throughout the process only makes the patient's experience and rehabilitation that much better.

Communication between all the people who are taking care of the patient is of utmost importance. Allied healthcare workers are in the trenches, working with the patient's temporary and long-term disabilities spiritually, physically, mentally, and emotionally. They keep the physician updated of the patient's progress, or lack thereof. They also notice other emotional or motivational issues that, when brought to my attention, greatly help me ensure the patient gets the maximal result.

I can still remember a time early in my practice when I had the opportunity to work with an occupational therapist (OT) whose office was adjacent to mine—actually, her door opened up into my office. I'm a fellowship-trained, hand-and-upper-extremities surgeon, and 50 percent of my work involves the hand and upper extremities. This OT/hand therapist was not only helpful but essential to maximizing care. When I would have a difficult patient, I'd ask her to come over and see the patient with me. Many times we would host a hand clinic where we would examine patients together in the office and brainstorm about their care. Once we came to a treatment decision, she would then take the patient next door to her office to attend to his therapeutic needs. We learned a lot from each other, but best of all, the patient received the highest level of compassionate care, communication, and understanding. I cannot remember a time when my patients got better care, all because of aligning with the right professionals to get the best results.

However, there's another member of the care team who may be the most important of all: the patient. If I do a complicated hand surgery like a flexor tendon repair, for example, I first need a motivated patient who will follow instructions and religiously do his therapy. My job as a surgeon includes not only performing the surgery with masterful skill and precision, but communicating my expectations to the patient, explaining what he will need to do to achieve a great result. I discuss with all my patients, prior to surgery, that the procedure is a partnership involving my surgical care and their agreement to do the rehabilitation necessary after to achieve maximal results. We must establish a level of trust between us, so even if progress isn't rapid, the patient trusts my guidance and feels reassured and motivated to follow it in order to go from fear to healing. Many times I describe my relationship with my patients as a partnership. Half of it is what I do, and the other half is what the patient will do under my and other healers' direction. If I spend time, effort, and energy to explain the patient's role in his own healing, it will do two things: it will prepare him for what's to come, and it will hopefully allay his fears.

Second, in addition to a motivated patient, I need an excellent occupational therapist to explain the appropriate exercises over the next three months to obtain the best results. Without the therapist's ongoing guidance as a part of postoperative care, the patient will most certainly get a less-than-satisfactory result, which may require additional surgery to correct the failed repair.

If egocentric physicians can put their egos aside and look at the big picture, the patient's care will unfold like a play where everyone in the play has an integral part—including the patient.

When it comes to finding the right team members for patient care, I have found a caring personality can mean more than years of experience. A newly trained nurse named Tracie attended to my mother during her last days, as she was in the hospital dying of lung cancer. She was wonderful, compassionate, and comforting to my mother as well as to our family. Even in the last hours before she passed, my mother felt and acknowledged the care that was present. Thanks to Tracie, those few days of hospice care in the hospital that ended in my mother's demise were tolerable.

A couple of weeks after my mother's death, my nurse retired, and I needed someone great to work for me. I thought of Tracie and contacted her to see if she had any interest in becoming my orthopedic nurse. She told me that she had little orthopedic experience, but I reassured her that I could teach her what she needed to know. She accepted the job, and for the next four years before I left the Midwest to move to California, we worked together side by side. She became an amazing assistant, and my patients were blessed by her care. Our team worked together like poetry in motion. I consider myself quite lucky to have been able to work with her. She still remains close as an adopted member of our family, even though we now live thousands of miles apart.

My nurse, medical assistant, physician's assistant, and appoint-ment/surgery scheduler are essential to the success of our patients' experience. If the patients are greeted by a helpful, caring appointment scheduler who gets them to the right specialist, the care starts off on the right track. After that, excellent communication needs to transpire between the other personnel. Any questions need to be answered, and medications, tests, and procedures need to be coordinated in a timely and helpful fashion. I remember changing dentists simply because his receptionist was not friendly or helpful when I tried to make an appointment. One of the most effective ways to sabotage your practice is to ask your patients to contact you with any questions and then not respond in a timely manner. Remember that the office personnel who interact with the patient before, during, and after surgery or treatment are also responsible for the care experience and keeping the patient happy, satisfied, and free of fear.

12. ADDRESSING PERSONALITY DIFFERENCES IN PATIENTS AND PHYSICIANS

Whenever the art of medicine is loved, there is also a love of humanity.

Hippocrates

As a group, physicians are rather diverse. My wife chuckles when she meets a group of physicians, because within a couple minutes of conversation, she can usually predict each one's particular subspecialty. Surgeons and ER docs are risk takers and will be the first to go after the adrenaline rush one gets from taking care of an acute trauma. In my case, that adrenaline rush comes by jumping out of a helicopter to get fresh tracks of snow. Nothing is more exhilarating than skiing through an incredibly steep powder field, and it's something I thoroughly enjoy. Most orthopedists are usually pushing the fitness edge and many times are being treated by their colleagues for their own injuries. Internists and cardiologists are much more conservative, diet conscious, and straight laced. Neurologists and pathologists are detail oriented and sometimes, respectfully, a little nerdy. The list goes on.

Many physicians practice medicine based on their interests and personality. A radiologist or anesthesiologist spends more time on his skill set and less time on patient communication. On the other hand, an internist or oncologist may spend extensive time working with the patient and family to affect a treatment or cure. A pediatrician practices by looking for clues to diagnose an illness in a patient that, many times, is less than communicative. No one specialty is better than another, and patient care is the primary focus of them all.

I'm happy to say I have been involved in the leadership of my multi-specialty group, and part of our leadership training involves something we call the leader lab. The leader lab includes psychological testing we take ourselves as well as peer evaluations by those we work with, which are completed and tabulated prior to the lab. As a result, one gets placed into a certain personality profile. My two-day lab experience included a group of about thirty different physicians and allied health personnel who all had different personality types.

On the first day, we did an exercise that put each of us into one of two groups: empathetic personality types and factual/technologically-oriented personality types. I was in the empathetic group. Each group was then asked to describe a picture that included three guys and a girl on a backyard deck. Our group described the picture as follows: one guy was feeling angry and left out, while the other three were good friends, enjoying each other's company. The other group described the picture as follows: they saw three Caucasian males—two wearing khaki pants and one wearing black shorts—and one Caucasian female wearing a tan dress, all on a brown-stained wooden deck. We were blown away. It was amazing to realize how differently different personalities can see the world. For the next few days, we worked together in small groups and discovered how our different personality types could best communicate and problem solve together. The experience was quite rewarding, but it also caused me to think about how we interact with our patients.

I know of many physicians' offices and groups that include short videos from physicians on their websites, so patients can get a sense of each physician's personality and whether they could relate well with him or her. How much better could our care and communication be if we could also identify our patients' personality types from the beginning?

I have been working on an idea about how I think we can improve the physician/patient relationship based on personality types. We could simply add questions to our new patient questionnaires that would help us determine whether patients are, for example, introverts or extraverts, or empathetic or technological, based on questions from validated personality tests.

We could input that information into the electronic medical records, and the physician who sees each patient would have instant insight into his personality and know how to best communicate with him. After all, the needs and concerns of patients with different personality types can vary considerably. Patients with a more technical perspective may require a lot of statistical analysis presented to them before they feel comfortable proceeding with a treatment. In contrast, more active decision makers may only require a simple presentation of the facts before they are ready to proceed with their treatment, without thinking twice.

However, most physicians don't receive emotional, psychological, or personality training to help them communicate effectively with their patients. Fortunately, some medical schools are beginning to offer this kind of training, such as Dr. Rachel Remen's course, "The Healer's Art," at the University of California at San Francisco. This course, which teaches medical students about the process of grief and how to be caring, is now offered at more than eighty medical schools and, in my opinion, should be basic to all programs. Even without specific training in medical school, many of us have figured out how to communicate with different patient personalities over the years (particularly the empathetic types), but it may be more difficult for others. Training physicians about how best to manage different personality types would even further improve communication and understanding between physicians and patients, allowing us to remove any unfounded fears about an upcoming procedure or treatment.

Effective healing depends on effective communication and understanding from both the physician and the patient. If we understood each other better, just think how much better the care could be.

PART THREE

Healing Our Healthcare System

*The art of medicine consists in amusing the patient
while nature cures the disease.*

Voltaire

13. THE NEED FOR PATIENT ADVOCATES

If you want others to be happy, practice compassion.
If you want to be happy, practice compassion.

Dalai Lama

I have thought of a model for a patient advocate system within healthcare that I think could be quite exciting. I think someone with medical knowledge who is caring, compassionate, and focused on the patient is imperative. Focus involves knowing the patient's history inside and out. It involves an understanding of his emotional and physical state. It involves understanding his home and work environment. It also involves an intuition about his needs, desires, habits, and motivations. To have this focus, one needs to have the time necessary to spend with the patient, interviewing and examining him or her to acquire this understanding. Some physicians have a sixth sense about patients they meet and their needs in the short time they spend with them.

This instantaneous connection is probably an exception, though. Most wonderful physician/patient relationships take a lot of time, effort, and energy to develop. It can take years, if not decades. Although we're a little past the time of making house calls, I can understand how rewarding that must have been. As I mentioned before, we have many friends and family members who know they can simply show up on my doorstep after I get home from work and I'll be happy to take a look at their injury. It always makes me feel wonderful to help in this way, and it is even more wonderful that my wife is so understanding; she is the one who tells them when I'll be home and encourages them to stop by.

Also, I can't even count how many times I've helped direct my family, friends, and patients through the medical system for problems outside my specialty. I have also enjoyed researching friends and family's medical issues on their behalf, and even though it's not my specialty, I can usually find the right answers and help direct their care. All it really takes is perseverance, care, and compassion to help them find answers.

Serving as their advocate, or "quarterback," helps take away a patient's fear and anxiety. Making medical decisions can be very difficult if you don't understand this field of medicine we work in, and I do anything I can to help others feel confident they're making a good, solid decision. Knowing they're supported throughout the process helps patients shift from a negative, stressed energy state to a positive one. This helps tremendously with ultimate healing, in my opinion. We all need a quarterback, or advocate, to help direct and guide us when we're not sure what we need.

Unfortunately, today's doctors have little time to provide the extensive communication and comfort essential to a patient's healing. For that reason, I've come up with the concept of a patient advocate system that would provide healthcare support and bridge communication gaps to ensure the patient's needs are taken care of. Each patient would have a patient advocate who would function like a quarterback for that patient's care team. A patient advocate would be someone with medical knowledge who is solely focused on the patient. Advocates would need a basic understanding of illness and disease in order to know where to look for help with their patients' care. The process would begin with an in-depth interview to gain a full understanding of the patient's medical history, current physical and emotional state, home and work environment, needs, desires, habits, and motivations. A patient advocate could be someone who is focused on a much smaller subset of patients and who could, therefore, direct a patient to a primary care physician or specialist for his specific illness or problem.

The advocate could then track the treatment path while supporting the patient all the way until healing is achieved. This care could provide a full understanding of the patient and his issues, from his lifestyle to his medical diagnoses.

So who would be qualified to be a patient advocate? I think nurse practitioners, physician assistants, registered nurses, semi-retired or retired physicians, and social work professionals fit this category of medically experienced and patient-focused advocates. Let me give you an example. I have a close friend, Dave, who has been a mentor, past partner in San Diego, and confidant. When he was in his early seventies, he stopped being a surgical orthopedist and spent time seeing and evaluating orthopedic patients. He spent over a year helping me see patients and assisting in surgery for one week a month in his transition to retirement. In his mid-seventies, he retired, but he still wanted to work in the field of medicine. He decided he would start doing evaluations through social security to evaluate disability.

He works part time and enjoys his work. It keeps him stimulated, as he is knowledgeable and intelligent, and it keeps him involved in the world of medicine, to which he's devoted sixty years of his life. Someone like Dave could be a perfect patient advocate.

However, this is not to say the primary care physician can't play this role for the patient. Many of us have a wonderful relationship with our primary care physician, and that trust, understanding, and dedication should never be tampered with. However, when a patient has many issues or problems, and he's seeing multiple specialists, then it's hard for the busy primary physician to keep track of everything. That's where the patient advocate could step in. Having someone to coordinate between the primary and all the patient's specialists could only help propel the patient in the best direction.

Also, many physicians now have concierge practices that take very attentive care of just a small number of patients for an additional fee. The patient advocate system could also begin as a type of concierge service, although I would love to see this service provided for all patients—not just those who can afford a higher fee.

Patient advocates would need an extensive training program to educate them in all areas related to coordinating patient care.

This would include training in communication, compassion, empathy, and the psychology of grief and dying. Advocates would also need to be trained to network with primaries and specialists, obtain information about a patient's illness to direct preventive care, and monitor care and improvement.

Finally, they would need to be trained to understand how alternative care, such as meditation, holistic medicine, acupuncture, chiropractic, craniosacral therapy, and physical and occupational therapy could connect to their patients' care and well-being. For example, knowing the options available for treating a cancer patient, whether it's the appropriate chemotherapy drug treatment or an alternative choice, is imperative for their care.

The patient advocate would also need to be educated in the necessary alternative and preventive care to advise their patients on additional ways to decrease one's stress and illness potential. A person trained, or at least knowledgeable, in a myriad of healing alternatives gives the patient every possible option for good health. Physicians tend to get focused on their own area of expertise, and like a racehorse with blinders, they don't always see things peripherally. Approaching an illness from a number of possible vantage points is not only helpful but essential. The advocate could assist the physicians in keeping their eyes open and greatly assist in the effectiveness of their care.

Not only do advocates need education, but just as in any medical school or nursing school, advocates also need experience in those healing processes. They should be taught how to meditate, experience an acupuncture treatment, and work in a therapy group with cancer patients to get insights in compassion, anger, fear, and pain. It is also probably important for them to watch a complicated surgery. They could even try Chinese or holistic treatments for their ailments. Specialists from all of these areas need to help train them and let them experience the ultimate benefits. Most of the advocates will already have a basic medical knowledge, but it's still important to train them in the latest science and also test them, providing the certification needed to practice. There are plenty of experts individually lecturing and having seminars who could teach advocates their techniques.

Although the patient advocate would have a great deal of knowledge and training in all these important areas, what's just as important is that the patient knows someone cares enough about him to research all available options to produce the ultimate positive result. It's kind of like what I experienced with my mom when I was a kid. When I was sick, my mother was concerned, focused, and loving. She would always make chicken soup and have me sip it. Of course, as a questioning child, I would ask "How do you know this will help make me feel better?" She would usually answer, "It won't hurt." You know what? It always made me feel better. Whether or not the soup had any inherent healing quality is a moot point. What really helped was the love and caring behind the giving.

A patient advocate system could be incorporated into our healthcare system in a number of different ways: it could be part of a government-subsidized system or a benefit provided through an insurance company. I have no doubt it would help to lower healthcare costs and diminish some of the defensive medicine practiced today, such as ordering excessive or inappropriate tests. A patient advocate could ensure the patient engages the healthcare system effectively and efficiently.

I hope this idea of a patient advocate system sparked your own ideas about how to improve our healthcare systems. Getting the best minds in one place to work together and develop a comprehensive approach to healing is just what the world needs. Just the thought of it is exciting and empowering. It's long past due, and our growing understanding of science, quantum physics, the power of compassion and love, and metaphysics can only help advance our capacity for healing further than our wildest dreams.

The future of healthcare depends on redesign, and ideas like the patient advocate system are part of that redesign. Understanding our patient population and their needs is part of that redesign. We need to bring compassion training back into medical training programs. Healers must once again become unconditionally dedicated to the Hippocratic Oath, and we must cast away the dogma that health professionals need to be strong instead of emotional or "touchy feely." Together, as patients and physicians, we need to lobby for the right things in Washington. Many politicians, including President Obama, have advocated for healthcare reform, but we all need to work together to make it happen in a way that produces the best healing result.

14. INTEGRATING EASTERN AND WESTERN MEDICINE

A generous heart, kind speech, and compassion are the things that renew humanity.

Buddha

I'm a huge advocate of combining the principles of Eastern and Western medicine to obtain maximal results. I first became acutely aware of the positive effects of Eastern medicine early in my collegiate career. I can still remember visiting with my good friend David in the early 1970s after he got back from a trip to China. I was a pre-med college student, and David was in his first year of an innovative six-year medical program in the Midwest.

As part of their curriculum, these students visited China to see how different medical care could be. I found the Chinese physicians' use of acupuncture to be particularly amazing. David came back from his trip with acupuncture needles and models of the ear and foot with marked areas for needle insertion, which correlated with certain areas of the body that could be anesthetized. He told me a fascinating story about a person who needed to have his gallbladder removed.

The surgery was performed in a large surgical suite that students could view from a glassed-in seating area above. The patient apparently walked in, bowed to the observers, and then was asked to lie down on the operating room table. He was prepped and draped, and then a couple of Chinese acupuncturists inserted needles in multiple areas in his ears and feet and began twirling them to anesthetize the area of surgery. The surgeon made a skin incision with the patient awake and removed the gallbladder.

After the wound was closed and dressed, the patient got off the table. Once again, he bowed to the observers and walked out of the operatory. The story was utterly amazing, yet true. As amazing as it was to hear about it, it was probably even more amazing for David and his class to observe it in person. At that point, I knew there was more to healing than traditional Western medicine. Simply understanding and being open to all forms of healing allows for infinite possibilities.

This reminds me of a funny story. I met my wife on a blind date. She was an international model and had lived all over the world, and as a result, was quite worldly.

We knew very little about each other, and I thought I could get to know her by taking her to see a baseball game. In the process of our discussion, after an hour or two, she finally asked what I did. I told her I was a surgeon, and her reaction was, "Oh, that's too bad."

When I asked why, she informed me that she didn't care too much for Western medicine or physicians, and she was very aligned with Eastern medicine. She had lived in several different countries overseas, so she had been exposed to many types of medical care, both traditional and non-traditional. She also had allergies to many antibiotics and had not had the best experience with Western medicine.

Of course, being totally infatuated with her mind and her beauty, I countered by saying that I believed in Eastern medicine also. She was quite surprised, but she now had more interest in me and there was potential for a relationship. Little did she know that at that time, my idea of Eastern medicine was something like a physician practicing medicine on the East Coast. In actuality, her eagerness and my openness changed my whole perspective on my approach to medicine. She helped to open my eyes to all the possibilities for caring for my patients, and together we have explored many alternative healing practices with our own maladies.

We have a multitude of alternative forms of healthcare available to us outside of traditional Western medical protocols and multitudes of forms within each specialty. Acupuncturists use their skills for anesthesia and pain control and also for healing the mind and the body. I can't even begin to name all the different forms of chiropractic medicine and its variations. Nowadays, it appears that the only major difference between osteopathic (DO) and medical (MD) training is that osteopathic training teaches you manipulation techniques to open up the blood and nerve connections from the spine to the extremities, which makes perfect sense, even if it's not a mandatory teaching subject anymore in osteopathic medical schools.

Natural and organic treatments, including a variety of Chinese and Indian herbs and treatments, are often safer than and just as (or more than) effective as typical pharmaceuticals. Many of these treatments have existed for centuries, and their recent resurgence indicates that we need an alternative approach to Western medicine, at least in some cases. When the treatment is worse than the disease, something has to change. Of course, all these alternative options also include some quackery and manipulation by some of the providers.

Whatever healing choice you make, be sure the clinical trials show its efficacy. I would be much more willing to take a harmless herb or other substance if it has been shown to be helpful than take some expensive drug with potential harmful side effects. As it is now, I rarely take much of anything. For me, the combination of a healthy diet, exercise, and preventive care has been the best approach for ongoing health.

Based on my experience, I have found several alternative forms of care to be particularly powerful and promising: meditation, energy healing, exercise, and a healthy diet.

MEDITATION

I am a huge advocate of using meditation to help calm one's mind, reduce stress, and re-energize. My wife and I have attended several of Deepak Chopra's seminars, as well as one of his meditation weeks, and during that process, we learned a lot about the tremendous health benefits of meditation and staying at a positive energy place. For example, according to quantum physics, everything we encounter, whether animate or inanimate, is energy. Meditation helps to stabilize and focus that energy at the highest possible state of vibration.

In her book *Train Your Mind, Change Your Brain*, Sharon Begley cites some excellent studies that compared patients with depression who used mindful meditation as a treatment and patients who took antidepressants. To simplify the results for the sake of discussion, those who meditated did just as well as those who took the medicine. Also, when the medicine was withdrawn, many patients had rebound depression, while those who stopped their meditation did not.[1] That's just one small example of the tremendous effects meditation can have on one's health, mind, body, and soul.

I have already alluded to the importance of approaching life from a state of positive energy. Putting good intentions out into the universe and then letting go of the outcome allows great things to transpire in our lives. Things are always much easier to digest with honey than with bitters. If you come from a loving, nonreactive place and do not let your ego get involved with the result of any interaction, your life will be enriched. Pouring out your best intentions to others and the universe, without expecting something in return, will result in more satisfaction and even a bit of serenity.

Being in a state of gratitude is imperative for happiness. Whether a circumstance appears positive or negative, you can always learn something from the experience, so in effect, every circumstance is positive in some way. You have to just be patient and trust that there is a grand design from a higher power. Plus, your positivity can affect others around you as

---

1   Sharon Begley, *Train Your Mind, Change Your Brain: How a New Science Reveals Our Extraordinary Potential to Transform Ourselves* (Ballantine, 2007).

well. If you doubt me, try this little exercise. Go out into the world and be as antagonistic, controlling, narcissistic, ego-based, and self-pitying as you can. Now, do you enjoy living a life where you're only looking out for yourself?

Or, if you know anybody who already lives like that in one form or another, step back and ask yourself: are they truly happy? Do they fare well in life? Are they gratified? Do they have wonderful and meaningful relationships? Have they achieved a sense of true serenity or enlightenment? I can assure you that living your life from a loving, compassionate, and unconditionally giving place is the primary path to true serenity, happiness, and enlightenment. You only have to try the alternative to believe it.

ENERGY HEALING

Everything we see and encounter in life is made of energy vibrating at different frequencies. Many energy practitioners who know how to focus energy in a positive way have achieved extraordinary things, including healing. Energy healers, craniosacral therapist, Reiki practitioners, and other trained energy healers abound, and their transformational work can have profound, life-changing effects when focused and done properly.

I have received some energy training and have seen its beneficial effects. I have done work on others using some of these techniques, and I have been worked on by other practitioners. Most practitioners of Western medicine have not been exposed to it and, as a result, may not be open to using energy healing as adjunctive care. I would challenge my medical colleagues who have not been exposed to it to try it on any of their own issues—the benefits may be eye opening. With more holistic approaches to the patient as a whole, the benefits of this hopefully will be used more commonly in the future. Being able to focus energy in a positive manner helps reduce stress and fear and aids in healing.

I personally have always known the power of positive energy. When my wife would have an ailment or discomfort, she would often ask me to place my hand on her sore elbow or shoulder. After gently placing my hand there or lightly massaging her area of injury, she would usually feel much better. As time went on and I became more aware of the positive effects of healing energy, I would focus more and more of my energy on the area of discomfort. Using the touch of my hands to focus the energy seemed helpful.

A few years ago, we took a vacation to Peru. When we were visiting Cusco, a place of intense energy, we decided to partake in a traditional ceremony with a local shaman. After the first part of this beautiful ceremony, we all went to different parts of the shaman's property to spend some time meditating. As the shaman walked by my wife, my wife noticed that she was in pain. The shaman had had recent surgery for a ruptured appendix and was having severe abdominal cramping to the point that she could hardly walk. My wife told her that I could probably help her, because I did healing with my hands.

The shaman came over to the area where I was meditating and told me she was in pain, indicating where the pain was. I asked her to lie down next to me. I placed my hand on her area of intense pain, and with all the energy I had, I focused on that area with all the positive intent I could muster. The result was an experience so intense that I found myself sweating and eventually had tears running down my cheeks. It was unlike anything I had ever experienced.

Within twenty minutes, the shaman got up, said her pain was gone, and told me that I was a powerful healer. As she walked away, I was astounded that I had the capacity to change a physical state by compassionately focusing my energy and positive intent on her ailment. I was grateful to have had the experience, knowing that I had ways other than using my surgical skills to aid my patients' health.

Surgeons tend to get quite focused on using their surgical skills alone to cure. Yes, a focused physician can achieve amazing things. It is how we were trained. We look at a problem and come up with a medical or surgical solution. But the cure requires more than just the technical fix. Many other things affect a patient's physical and emotional state. I try to approach everyone I encounter from a place of positive energy, especially those I'm treating. I try my best to calm their fear through compassionate communication and try to give my full attention to the patient—when I first meet them, before surgery, and after surgery. As I mentioned earlier, I have spent time understanding the different personality types, and as a result, I am better able to communicate in a way patients can understand. I frequently use humor as an adjunct to dissipate anxiety and calm any fear. Any time the patient stays in a scared or anxious place, it's hard to achieve maximal healing. Dissipating their fear and having a positive perspective creates trust, and the patient can't help but get better.

I also believe in positive energy healing. Now, when I talk to a patient before their surgery, I usually take their hand in mine or place my hand on their injured extremity and, without them knowing that I'm focusing my energy through touch, I tell them not to worry and to let me do the worrying. I ask them to visualize using their repaired knee or shoulder, for example, with no pain after their procedure is done.

That interlude helps me project my positive energy to that person, and the visualization, touch, and compassionate dialogue energizes my patients as well as myself. I am blessed by the fact that I have had very few surgical issues or complications, and I hope it has everything to do with my skill, caring, and approach.

DIET AND NUTRITION

I can't stress enough the importance of a healthy diet. Our general population is overweight and out of shape. Our diets are filled with artificial sweeteners, corn-fed and steroid-laden meats, and fast food. On the other hand, the right foods have antioxidants that can help fight infection, cancer, and heart disease. Nutritionally, organic foods of most types are better for you and have less potential to cause disease or infections. Fortunately, permaculture and growing our own food as a community has become an undeniable movement. There's hardly a city anymore that doesn't have a farmers market where you can buy fresh, organic produce. Documentaries like *Food, Inc.* and *Super Size Me* have opened our eyes to the deleterious effects of foods whose purpose is to profit the company instead of nutritionally enriching the recipient.

Unfortunately, it's significantly cheaper for people to buy the foods that are nutritionally deficient than the ones that are actually good for you. Studying the labels is a good first step to determine if the foods are nutritious and organic. More and more healers and physicians are focused on diet and nutrition, and extensive resources are available (beyond the scope of this book to cover). If you are concerned with your health as you should be, you should confer with your healer or nutritionist to help guide you toward a healthier lifestyle.

Here too, traditional Eastern practices can educate and enlighten us. Ayurvedic teaching involves connecting the mind and body to heal and transform the body. An Ayurvedic diet consists of fresh, organic foods balanced among the six major tastes—sweet, salty, sour, pungent, bitter, and astringent—and the colors of the rainbow. Of course, as we know now, purple, blue, red, orange, or green foods are usually high in antioxidants and contain many nutrients that boost health and immunity. As Ayurvedic teaching advises us, when one combines meditation, yoga, and a holistic approach to illness with a natural or Ayurvedic diet (one based on traditional Indian practice), wonderful things begin to happen.

EXERCISE

What has happened to the days I remember as an adolescent, when every Saturday you'd run out the door after breakfast and play outside with friends in the neighborhood until you heard your mother calling your name to come home for dinner? Today, we've become a population of computer nerds, video gamers, and TV watchers who aren't doing even basic exercise. Exercise is so important for one's physical and mental health. Exercising helps the heart, keeps the bones strong, reduces stress, and increases the levels of circulating endorphins that affect pain receptors and centers of well-being in the brain. Yoga has the added benefit of combining stretching, exercise, and meditation.

I'm an every-day exerciser. I am much more productive, calm, and clear thinking, with a general sense of well-being, when I exercise regularly. In fact, I feel like a grouchy, impatient, sluggish guy when I don't work out. The list of benefits goes on and on. Personally, exercise and meditation are my cornerstones. They allow me to achieve the balance needed in a busy surgeon's life.

In particular, I am a long-time runner. I'm sure many of you have heard about a runner's high. It's that high level of circulating endorphins achieved during a run that takes the runner to an almost meditative or Zen-like state. It allows the runner to clear his mind and propels him down his path. I know it happens in many other sports as well. For me, after the initial elevation of my heart rate and endorphins, I find myself transported to a meditative and calm place. As my mind clears, I have epiphanies about my life. My senses observe nature more keenly. It's an incredible calm and comforting place, much like the state I experience when I meditate. It is truly the only thing I know that allows me to get rid of my daily stresses.

I can't adequately stress the importance of exploring other alternative treatments. Yoginis, Zen masters, and Ayurvedic teachers have spent their lifetime studying and living these older ways. Even the laws of Kashrut (or Kosher laws) recorded in the Talmud were dietary laws based on what was appropriate for sustaining health. For example, many people know that not eating pork is one of the principles of keeping kosher. Only later did we discover that centuries ago, poorly cooked pork contained the trichina worm, which was detrimental to one's health.

I believe incorporating alternative care into our definition of healing is foundational to our healthcare system. Medical schools need to educate new physicians about effective, evidence-based preventative and alternative care practices so they can include them in their diagnostic and referral process. Continuing education about alternative care for particular specialties could be offered more widely as well. Just as physicians have a responsibility to provide the best care for their patients, patients have a responsibility to take charge of their own health through basic preventative practices like diet, exercise, and stress management. That way they don't have to rely on their healthcare provider to treat the inevitable diseases that result from poor eating choices, a sedentary lifestyle, and stress. Also, patients can start taking advantage of alternative care such as meditation and energy healing right now; information on these practices has never been more abundant. If both physicians and patients include preventative and alternative care practices in their definitions of healthcare, imagine how it would streamline healthcare costs and treatment time.

Everyone's approach to life is different, but I would encourage all to keep their mind and eyes open to different forms of alternative care. Combining Eastern and Western medical principles, and adopting a mindset of approaching life from a loving place, can't help but make us healthier and happier.

15. THE INSURANCE INDUSTRY

If insurance companies paid for lifestyle-management classes, they would save huge sums of money. We need to see that alternative medicine is now mainstream.

Deepak Chopra

Patient autonomy is paramount to the oath that we take when we enter the profession of medicine. That is why I am appalled when the federal government gets between my patients and their right to the full range of medical information and complete access to healthcare.

Ami Bera

We all know major issues are hindering the effectiveness of our healthcare system. The entire system is long past due for a shift from a greed-motivated system that generates mistrust and fear to a healing-motivated system that generates trust. As a physician, I see three major problem areas: the insurance industry, the legal industry, and the pharmaceutical industry. The lobbying in Washington for these three industries is powerful, and these lobbies have limited our ability to provide excellent healthcare for this country. Unfortunately, as healthcare providers, our focus is not usually on our political system. Although there have been some recent attempts to correct these problems, as of now, I don't believe these efforts have been very successful. I perceive greed to be a primary motivator, and it's frustrating to sit back and watch attempts to fix the system without very much potential for success. You all know these problems as well as I do and have experienced them firsthand.

I've watched the Democrats and the Republicans argue over healthcare reform. President Obama has begun to try, with inadequate results, to help correct our insurance system's deficiencies. The politicians' focus is entirely in the wrong place. Money is made from our patients, and the majority of the profits go into the pockets of corporate executives. Their selfish and greedy motives hold us back and limit our ability to have the best, most caring, most successful system in the world. Hopefully, with the right focus—on healing—we can achieve that in the future.

Without a doubt, our healthcare system in the United States needs to be better integrated, with politicians, physicians, insurance companies, and corporations all working in concert to keep the focus on what's truly in the best interest of patient care. A win-win situation for the patient, physician, healthcare professional, insurance company, and corporation can happen—if everyone is willing to work together. Our government wants to take on the responsibility of regulating the medical world, which is understandable. What would work best, however, is if we could regulate ourselves.

I am not a political guy. I don't profess to have the knowledge to come up with a plan to correct the federal deficit, stop global warming, or prevent terrorism. But I do have some valid views about our healthcare system after spending the last thirty-four years practicing medicine, and I bet some of my colleagues do too. Even though I am open for suggestions on how best to impact these three industries, I do have some firm ideas about what needs to change. Let's begin with our insurance industry.

Our country, as great as it is, still lacks the ability to provide healthcare for all. If 15 percent of our country is without healthcare, then it is 15 percent too many. Some physicians go to third-world countries and donate their time and medical and surgical expertise. I think being charitable in that fashion is wonderful. Unfortunately, we still have problems in our own country. We have a significant percentage of our population who don't have insurance coverage or can't afford the insurance.

Before we run off to other places, it might be good if we take care of our own needs at home first. One solution to caring for the uninsured and indigent could be to require all physicians to provide community care to the poor and indigent or uninsured as part of board certification or re-certification requirements. We haven't been able to rely on the insurance companies to help with this problem, but perhaps we can engage our specialty boards to work directly with government agencies.

This would be nothing more than our responsibility to others as part of the Hippocratic Oath. It would, without a doubt, be much more effective if we could engage physicians, insurance companies, and politicians to work as a team to come up with a way to provide healthcare for all, in the best interest of all. Again, I'm not a politician or an insurance executive. I am merely a physician offering my opinions from a place of rational common sense, seeking the best interest of my patients.

Imagine a world where insurance companies were in a competitive environment to provide unrestricted healthcare, a place where there were no preexisting health restrictions on care and every individual had access to the healthcare he needed. It would be great if a patient wouldn't have to worry about his high deductible and could simply ilicit help for his medical issues. Patients now tend to hold off on getting care because the deductibles have gone through the roof to cover previously excluded insurance costs. Unfortunately, in our current United States model, insurance companies and their lobbies have been a major factor in driving up the cost of medicine.

An insurance company that pockets profits by blocking authorization for x-ray tests, medical or surgical care, or medicine for a patient's arthritis, hypertension, or cancer puts both the patient and the physician at risk. When a system provides care but the insurance company denies and delays access to and payment for that care, the patient suffers financially, physically, and emotionally. When companies exclude preexisting medical conditions, such as cardiac issues, it's a travesty, and it's hard not to interpret it as greed.

As we'll discuss further in the next chapter, when the patient gets a poor result due to this withholding of care, he wants to sue his physician *and* his insurance company. Plenty of hungry attorneys help drive up the malpractice premiums for the physician, which further encourages the practice of "defensive medicine." Physicians coming from a place of fear or insecurity order more tests, sometimes unnessarily, which results in overcharging for their visits and care. All of this, in addition to diminishing insurance reimbursements, creates a vicious cycle that works directly against excellence in patient care.

Patients need to advocate for more comprehensive medical care without restrictions, and physicians need to be on the bandwagon supporting them. When I have a patient who needs a treatment, therapy, or a test during my care that isn't covered, I get incensed. I'll be the first to write a letter on the patient's behalf to urge the company to extend benefits, and I'll be happy to call an insurance gatekeeper and give him a piece of my mind.

I can remember recently seeing a patient with a torn meniscus in her knee. She had previously been in another healthcare system, and after three months of pain, her insurance company finally authorized an MRI to diagnose the condition, which was when her meniscus tear was identified. She was now on a three- to four-month waiting list to get her arthroscopic surgery. Then her health insurance changed, and I was now a covered provider. So she came to see me as a new patient and showed me her MRI findings. After my exam, she asked when I could perform her surgery.

I can still remember the look of disbelief on her face when I replied, "Next week." I'm a very busy surgeon, but I still had time to fit her procedure in because it was in her best interest. It was a simple arthroscopic surgery that takes about forty-five minutes of surgery time.

Her care had been delayed so long because, prior to switching insurance companies and seeing me, she had been part of an insurance system that provided cheaper coverage (although it was the most she could afford) and failed to prioritize her procedure. The delay kept her in pain, limited her ability to work, and impacted the quality of her life. In the same way, when an insurance company delays authorization for initiating cancer treatment, that delay may allow it to spread, possibly diminishing any chance for a cure. These insurance decisions are certainly not made for the patient's best interest. Regardless of your insurance carrier, a big delay in treatment should not be allowed to occur.

If the government does anything, it would be great if it could legislate restrictions on what insurance companies can or cannot do. These situations border on criminal neglect. Lobbies abound to protect the best interest of the politicians and corporations, but healthcare needs to be for the best interest of the patient. When we lose sight of the patient, we lose sight of medicine. Without the patient, healthcare doesn't exist.

Another insurance reform needed involves how insurance companies deal with physicians. Many companies hold physicians hostage with their reimbursement tactics. They lure you in with promises of what they will pay for your service in an HMO or PPO program. Soon after, as a cash-saving approach to maximize the company's profit, they start restricting what you can order and, worse, what they will reimburse you for your care. The small medical group is squeezed when told, "Even though last year we reimbursed you sixty cents on the dollar, we now can only reimburse you forty-five cents."

If the small group protests, the insurance company usually threatens it with losing the opportunity to take care of that patient. If the small group doesn't like it, the insurance company replaces it with another medical group. As a result, the group either has to accept the lower reimbursement and see more patients in the same amount of time or increase their charges to cover costs and overhead. The patient suffers from less efficient care at higher prices, which also pushes up the cost of healthcare.

I feel blessed to be part of a large healthcare organization/ multi-specialty group that has businessmen negotiate these contracts and help the group to stand up to the insurance company's squeeze. When an insurance company tells a big, multi-specialty group that it will be reimbursed less under the new terms of their contract, and the group says, "Okay, we'll just withdraw our coverage for hundreds of thousands of patients," I can assure you that the insurance group will think twice. It's a shame that it comes down to this, but unfortunately, that's our reality. The real question is, what is the objective of the health insurance company? Shouldn't their mission be to provide the opportunity to get excellent care and treatment?

Let's look at a more intricate patient care scenario to show how insurance companies can contribute to the delay and/ or hinder the ultimate achievement of healing. Let's say John Doe gets into an accident either on the road, in his car, or at work. He's brought to the hospital unconscious, and after weeks of ICU care, surgeries, and extensive tests, he's ready to go home. He is battered, bruised, and disabled. He's trying to heal from his ordeal with a positive attitude and with help from wonderful healers. Then, he gets a bill for an inordinate amount, possibly hundreds of thousands of dollars. Now the fight begins.

His health insurance blocks further care and won't pay his medical bills, saying the accident was work related or their payment should be secondary in an accident where there is another party responsible. If it was work related, the workers' comp group may want him to go to a different doctor, and as a result, the continuity of care is interrupted. If the other driver was at fault in the accident, then the insurance company may demand that the other party involved in the accident cover the cost. A legal battle may ensue over who is responsible for the care and payment for the bills. The patient can't work, has bills to pay, might lose his job, and has a huge debt that might affect his credit negatively. He's now in the middle of a lot of negatives, instead of being in a positive place as he tries to heal.

The stress from his injury and the aftermath is overwhelming. Many patients in this scenario ultimately have to get an attorney to sort it out. This again adds more cost and stress to the patient and delays his care. The patient will ultimately have problems getting well until the case is resolved. A legal battle could take years for resolution. This all-too-typical situation has great psychological, physical, and legal ramifications. In an environment like this, it is hard to get well.

I can personally attest to how insurance companies can maneuver around payment for services. My wife recently was having a spell of headaches, which subsequently resolved. She saw her primary care physician, and he suggested getting an

MRI of her brain. Luckily, it was normal. The interesting part is that even though I'm a physician who is part of a large, multi-specialty group that farms its insurance out to an outside company, I received a bill for twenty-five hundred dollars. I waited for a while, checking my monthly medical bill to see if it had been paid. After three months of seeing that charge on my bill, I decided to call the company instead.

The insurance call center guided me through a series of prompts, and finally, after about twenty minutes, I got to speak to an actual person about my bill. When I questioned the billing representative about why the MRI wasn't covered by my insurance, she asked if we answered the questionnaire sent to us about the nature of my wife's problem. Apparently they needed to know more about the nature of my wife's problem and whether it happened from an accident. We never received a questionnaire, nor did we receive a call from the insurance company. In reality, the company was simply delaying payment. I believe they were hoping I would just pay the recurring bill before it affected my credit or was sent to collections. Perhaps they hoped some other insurance company would cover the cost if this was related to an accident.

I honestly felt scammed. How many times had I paid past bills that the insurance company should have covered? The coverage is often confusing, and the bills just keep on coming. Sometimes it's easier to pay the bill than take the time to research the coverage or actually make contact with an insurance representative.

These tactics cause a great deal of stress and frustration. How can someone really get well and heal with all these financial worries that too often ensue after an illness or injury? I'm not saying all health insurance systems are less than legitimate. Many do the right thing. But it would be nice if most of us didn't feel like we were a character in the movie *Erin Brockovich,* when all the insurance companies are processing claims and requests with deny, deny, and deny!

I believe at least part of the solution to this dilemma is for insurance companies to provide unrestricted coverage for all care—not just for injuries and illnesses but (especially) for preventative care. Let the insurance companies, which we all pay our premiums to, have their own legal or workers' comp department deal with who gets to pay for what. That would leave the patient with no worries except whatever it takes to get well. When the patient is concerned about how to pay for or get the care he needs for treatment, he's already behind the eight ball.

Further, if the insurance plan has a huge deductible of five thousand to ten thousand dollars, the patient may never see a practitioner for routine preventative care or even obvious needs, causing delays in treatment that may dramatically affect his health.

With all the premiums we pay to insurance companies, surely we can afford another part of the solution: to reasonably reimburse the physician. When the physician's costs are not adequately covered, the patient's care will also suffer, and the numbers of excellent physicians available will decrease as they get disenchanted with the practice of medicine.

Many politicians, like Ted Kennedy, Bill and Hillary Clinton, and President Barack Obama have tried to bring about systemic change. They have tried to come up with a workable plan that seeks a cooperative political environment to remove the profit factor and provide compassionate care. But the most recent attempt, the Affordable Care Act, has many issues. Many who previously had more expensive plans have transitioned to a new plan, but unfortunately, they have encountered a startling reality. I have a friend and patient who recently changed her insurance under the Act to a PPO. After she switched and became ill, she discovered that she now has a huge deductible, could no longer see me or any of her other physicians—including her primary—and couldn't get in to see anyone else because schedules were full. When I inquired within my own group as to why we couldn't see her, I found out our group wasn't covered under the Act. What a travesty and so sad that the care she needed was delayed. It caused her incredible anxiety and fear, which adversely added to her illness. In this case, the Affordable Care Act was neither affordable, nor did it provide compassionate care.

Certainly, a lot more work needs to be done, and physicians and patients should be the ones driving the boat towards the best course of action. The attempts to engage physicians and insurance companies in working together have had less than satisfactory results. As physicians, we can probably come up with a way to serve the uninsured. We could also help design an insurance company business model that provides unrestricted care and trusts physicians and patients to come up with the best course of action. Once we have a workable business model, we can then engage our political system for support. There has to be a better way!

16. THE LEGAL SYSTEM

I think there is a sort of box-ticking mentality. Not just in the teaching profession. You hear about it in medicine and nursing. It's lawyer-driven insistence on meeting prescribed standards rather than just being a good doctor.

Richard Dawkins

My next major concern about healthcare lies with our legal system. I've already alluded to the damage to healing caused when legal issues delay care. If you can't get treatment or surgery because your payment hasn't been legally determined yet, patient care suffers. Again, I think the patient should be left out of the battle over who is responsible for paying and kept out of the process. Insurance companies should provide the same care for all, regardless of how the problem occurs.

If insurance companies are in the healthcare business, then they should use their resources to figure out where payment should come from, instead of padding their corporate bank accounts by delaying or denying care. The attorneys benefit as well and would love nothing more than to drag out the process with conferences, depositions, trials, and unlimited legal fees. Of course, the trial is just another part of the legal battle, which is costly and further delays care and healing. The battle over responsibility for payment of services has engaged the legal system, driving physicians to practice defensive medicine, which has driven up healthcare costs dramatically. (I know I sound critical of the legal and insurance systems. I do believe they each have their role, but I wish it could be done differently.)

In fact, defensive medicine is probably one of *the* greatest reasons for the rise in healthcare costs. From rising malpractice premiums to the ordering of excessive tests and scans, the costs have gotten out of control. The legal system, with and without tort reform, has put a lot of pressure on physicians, and when care doesn't turn out perfectly, physicians fear a lawsuit.

Many times the fear of missing something in our diagnosis or treatment pushes us to order additional tests or procedures. The additional test may be excessive or unnecessary, but it can be done out of a desire to best serve the patient.

For example, when a patient comes to see me, as an orthopedic surgeon, I almost always order x-rays. I figure that when they see me as a specialist, radiographs should be done to make sure there are no structural issues. I have backed off that premise somewhat because many times, in younger patients, basic films are relatively normal for patients without chronic pain. But if we miss something by not ordering or testing, the patient may suffer—and we may be facing some legal ramification. Even when our own radiologists see an x-ray with a small abnormality, they often suggest doing a more involved scan like a CT or an MRI to more clearly delineate a minimal abnormality on a plain x-ray.

As a specialist, when I see this, I feel compelled to order the more advanced tests because the radiologist suggested it. Many times the additional testing is normal, but the radiologist and the specialist are simply ordering it to cover their asses.

To be honest, the thought of being involved in litigation nauseates me. In my three-decade career in medicine, I've only been named in two lawsuits. Both suits named everyone involved with the patient's care, whether they took care of the patient to the best of his ability or not. Luckily, I was dropped from the litigations, along with many others, but not before I went through the agony and anxiety of the entire process. If a physician gets sued, he has to undergo a process that involves expensive litigation involving depositions, attorney meetings, and court appearances. I can tell you from experience that the process is always in the back of one's mind—even causing physicians to wake up regularly in a cold sweat at two in the morning. The anxiety and stress from an impending litigation that could last for a year or two makes your gut turn over on a regular basis. I had to do a chart review, discuss my care with an attorney, set up a defense, and then wait until I either had to go to court or was dismissed from the lawsuit. What an emotional waste of time and money for everyone!

Most of us do a lot of soul searching when we give our best effort, and even with that effort, we sometimes don't get the best results. Luckily my medical group has a wonderful risk management department, which I am part of, that evaluates problems that develop involving patient care. It helps guide and support us with this unfortunate process, whenever it occurs.

Whenever complaints arise from either physicians or patients, we internally make decisions about whether care was appropriate or the provider needs a reprimand. Many times we place physicians, if needed, on a physician improvement plan, and if they don't improve their care, they may be asked to leave. We are also self-insured for malpractice and have our own legal team if needed, so I believe we do a good job with our own risk management. As a result, our legal expenses are minimized as well as our group's exposure, which results in lower malpractice costs and excellence in patient care. This greatly helps to keep the costs of medicine down, particularly the need for the physician or caregiver to have to practice defensive medicine. If we could follow our practice's model on a widespread level, malpractice premiums would go down, as well as overall medical costs.

The majority of us practice with integrity and the best of intention. Being judged and criticized by a group of non-medical attorneys and the lay public on a jury is demeaning and painful. Many times malpractice companies push to settle a case, which tarnishes the physician's record, in order to save additional costs to the company by moving towards a trial. The attorney representatives first threaten a bigger settlement and punitive damages, as well as a bigger blemish to the physician's record, and then push to settle. Sometimes they can settle even without your consent, which leaves one even more incredulous.

Also, many times the physician is acting well within the standard of care. A new way to litigate, which can show up on physician's record, is to file a claim against a physician in small claims court. Many times a patient does this because he simply doesn't want to pay the bills. Even though the monetary limit is low, the claim is decided by a small claims court judge. This judge can decide a case without all the facts or legal representation, and it still blemishes a physician's record. Although there's been a huge push to improve patient satisfaction and mitigate patient complaints so as to avoid these kinds of nuisance suits, there has to be a better way.

A very small subset of physicians, whose primary motivation is to take advantage of the patient and the insurance system, have adversely affected the whole healthcare system. In the last twenty-five years, I have experienced only a few business-oriented physicians who were operating too aggressively. Unfortunately, some physicians are prioritizing wealth and profit over patient care. These doctors have made patients skeptical and have brought the attorneys out of the woodwork.

Many years ago, in my first practice setting, I was working with an associate who was a poor technician with a big ego. I wandered into the operating room while he was working on a young woman's knee. He was trying to remove a bone abnormality, which he could not find in his open wound. When I asked him what the problem was, he replied that he could not find the abnormality in the wound just below the knee. I went over to look at the abnormality on the x-ray view box and saw an L on the x-ray, which denoted the left knee. When I looked at the surgeon and the open wound, I saw he was working on the right knee. I was quite startled, but after I regained my composure, I asked the surgeon to walk over to the view box with me.

I quietly notified him that he was working on the wrong extremity. He cleaned up the right knee, closed the wound, and then prepped and draped the other leg. He then performed the procedure and closed the left leg. After the surgery was over, in the recovery room and on the floor, he told the patient that the operating personnel had made a mistake and prepped the wrong leg and unfortunately she had two incisions to heal. He did not take responsibility, and he placed the blame on someone else. As a result, the patient was livid. She refused to have this physician follow her in the hospital after that. Somehow, I was drafted to help console her and see her postoperatively.

The question is, did she sue him? The answer is yes, of course. If the surgeon would have been honest, communicated his mistake, taken responsibility, and apologized, maybe not. Fortunately, mistakes are very infrequent in hospital operating rooms and outpatient surgical centers now that surgeons and patients are constantly being questioned about what's being worked on. The patient and physician even have to mark the extremity or surgical site prior to surgery. Regardless, physicians like the example above negatively affect the whole healthcare system with their ego. Their actions run up the costs, and they need to be filtered out. However, I don't believe we need attorneys to police us; we can do it ourselves. I'll say more about that later.

In addition to creating fear about lawsuits and legal fees, the legal system also negatively affects our healthcare system by driving malpractice rates through the ceiling. Nowadays, it costs a lot to practice medicine. A physician in a small group or on his own has major financial stress from rising malpractice premiums and lower reimbursement for his care from insurance companies or Medicare. He tries to survive by seeing more patients and adding volume to his practice to make ends meet. He has his office overhead and staff to consider also. Again, I realize I'm quite fortunate to be part of a very large medical group that is self-insured. Our groups malpractice insurance covers us whether we are working as an employee or a shareholder, and we have a legal team that supports us.

In a big group, sometimes we lose some autonomy, but our costs are better covered. When a physician in a small group starts "churning," working overtime to see as many patients as possible to make ends meet, he can end up ordering excessive tests, and his communication with the patient—not to mention patient care itself—may suffer. I have known physicians who are so busy that they rarely perform a physical exam and rely on diagnosis based on laboratory and radiographic testing. This, to me, does not exemplify providing excellent medical care.

I'm concerned about the future of medicine. The anxiety of being involved in litigation and high malpractice rates may drive even an excellent physician out of practice or into early retirement. It can also persuade a gifted student not to choose medicine as a career. Most students are fairly savvy now and look at the cost of extensive education over many years and the loans they expect to incur before they generate earnings. It could easily be hundreds of thousands of dollars in loans before they're done. Before I could become a practicing orthopedic surgeon, I had to go through fourteen years of education and training after high school. For the first eight years, I had no income and for the next six years, just a small amount. It's hard to start practicing medicine at the age of thirty-five with huge incurred debt. In retrospect, I personally would do it all over again, but if one is not dedicated, the costs can seem to far outweigh the benefits.

At the end of the arduous journey of education and training, these prospective doctors, looking at low salaries and reimbursements, may also have to navigate through shark-infested legal waters—which could also make one question why he would want to go into medicine.

As I said earlier, I don't believe we need the legal system to police us. Most of us serve our patients with the best of intentions. We go through extensive training and have to satisfy requirements to get into medical school, graduate from medical school, and graduate from specialty training programs. Additionally, we have to satisfy oral and written examinations to obtain board certification. Every decade, we have to again satisfy similar requirements and be re-certified. Hospitals, surgical centers, medical groups, and the state boards have guidelines that monitor all of us who practice medicine.

If a doctor has a complication or problem that arises in the treatment of a patient, it often triggers the peer review process. Certain guidelines isolate problem cases, like readmission to a hospital within thirty days after discharge. If a problem is isolated, then the physician is required to present the case to a group his peers. The physician then gets feedback and constructive criticism, or perhaps accolades. We live in an imperfect world, and even with the best efforts, problems can occur. None of us are beyond reproach. Hopefully these evaluations screen out those physicians who do not care for their patients with the utmost integrity. I always say the best judge of one's character after one falls down is how he gets back up—what he tries to do to make it right.

A doctor giving his best effort is paramount to healing. If a physician is acting poorly or outside the standard of care, no one knows it better than his peers. They should be judge and jury and decide the consequences, whether it's a simple reprimand or suspension or the loss of one's license at the very extreme. Local problems can be relayed to state and specialty boards, which have their own additional peer review process. If the board reviews care that is deemed "outside the standard of care," the physician can be suspended or even lose his license. Many times there are legal ramifications from these actions and, of course, fear surrounding this entire process. I know that when my group evaluates a physician under the direction of the risk management team, a complete peer review is done. If they find multiple issues of unacceptable care and no chance for improvement, the physician is terminated.

Attorneys scrutinizing physicians are doing nothing more than driving up healthcare costs and physicians' malpractice costs. If our government wants to help bring down healthcare costs, let them set up laws and, even better, tort reform to limit settlements. I truly believe that we, as a profession, will do what's right.

17. THE PHARMACEUTICAL INDUSTRY

One of the first duties of the physician is to educate the masses not to take medicine.

William Osler

The pharmaceutical industry likes to depict itself as a research-based industry, as the source of innovative drugs. Nothing could be further from the truth. This is their incredible PR and their nerve.

Marcia Angell

The third industry negatively affecting the healthcare system is the pharmaceutical lobby. The rising cost of drugs is a definite factor contributing to our rising healthcare costs. The high cost of drugs cause insurance companies not to pay for certain medicines that patients need to keep their disease under control or affect a cure, and the out-of-pocket expense can be prohibitive—even while the same or similar drugs are much less expensive in other countries. People die every day because they can't afford the cost of treatment or get the drugs they need to keep their blood pressure under control or eradicate their cancer. If we're seeking the best of compassionate care, our patients shouldn't have to face this.

I was quite impressed when years ago I saw Michael Moore's movie called *Sicko*. In the very beginning of this movie, they interviewed an eighty-eight-year-old man mopping floors in the supermarket. I wasn't sure whether he was holding the mop or the mop was holding him up. In the interview, he was asked why he was still working at his age. He indicated that in his retirement, he had very limited monetary reserves, and his Medicare insurance didn't cover the cost of his expensive heart medications needed to keep him and his wife alive. Without the medication, he was sure they would die, and that was why he was still working.

The whole interview definitely had an emotional impact on me, but it reflected reality. The elderly on a limited income can't usually afford these medicines, and I've known people working into their eighties—those golden years—just to make enough money to pay for medication to keep them alive. The profits keep going into the pockets of the corporate executives and their shareholders, and the poor or elderly keep getting sicker. Situations like that are deplorable, and I wish our government would step in with some kind of new reform. Medicare Part D is supposed to cover medications, but it does so incompletely. We can do better to care for all, especially our elderly.

I have a friend who, after college graduation, worked for a nonprofit that raised money to help poor senior citizens pay for their medications. If they qualified, they got a card where they could pay a five dollar copay for medicines on the formulary, and they got many local drug stores and pharmacies to accept the card. There were also pharmacists on staff to do free medication reviews, which were mandatory every six months. Many of these elderly were on multiple medications with adverse drug interactions. She told me it was eye opening to see that many times multiple specialists attending to these elderly were prescribing drugs, but the doctors often didn't realize what other medications the patients were taking because the elderly couldn't remember it themselves. The good thing is there was at least a nonprofit group trying to improve this process, even if they encountered some challenges and roadblocks. The reality is that programs like this need to become our standard of care.

Insurance premiums, malpractice suits, and pharmaceutical costs are out of sight. All of us working together through blogs, forums, social media, and local meetings will help impact our legislation locally and in Washington. Our politicians are supposed to be "for the people," and I would challenge them to come forward on our behalf without a secondary agenda. If we can all work together from a place of compassion and integrity, our economy, healthcare, and healing energy would take us all to a place better than we could have ever imagined.

CONCLUSION: A VISION FOR COMPASSIONATE HEALTHCARE

Simplicity, patience, and compassion. These three are your greatest treasures.

Lao Tzu

Hopefully, our next question is, where do we go from here? I've tried to share with you the sometimes arduous journey a physician, holistic practitioner, or anyone in the allied health field has to take to get to a place where he can help to heal others. I've tried to stress the importance of how the physician needs to go from a place of ego, greed, and fear to a place of trust and compassion with his patients and those he takes care of. If it's done well, hopefully the patient's experience will change dramatically, and the patient can also shift from a place of fear to a place of trust and wholeness. Finally, I've tried to highlight what in the healthcare system could be changed to help promote the shift from fear to compassion for all. Hopefully I can now summarize what I believe it will take to transform healing and healthcare.

TRANSFORMING THE PHYSICIAN/PATIENT RELATIONSHIP

My role as a physician and surgeon comes with great responsibility, in that my decisions dramatically affect the lives of others. There is so much more to my job than just understanding the science, anatomy, surgical and medical treatment protocols, and the nuts and bolts of navigating the healthcare system. Our effectiveness is directly proportional to the balance we keep in our personal life and how we balance the lives of others. Dedicated professionals have to be able to put their ego and monetary gain on the back burner and make the best interest of their patients their primary focus. The patients are responsible for the software and the healers for the hardware. Keeping healthcare professionals focused on the right place is paramount to healing.

The more the healthcare professional gets exposed to the psychology of taking care of others and learns how to do this compassionately, the better our system will be. As I mentioned before, we are blessed with people like Dr. Rachel Remen, whose "Healer's Art" course has been incorporated in about eighty medical schools all over the world, thanks to her and her colleagues. As I've stated before, it's very frustrating as a surgeon and a physician who's been in practice for over three decades to watch newer physicians who are sometimes on a different healing trajectory and not focused on the patient first. I know how important it is to balance one's personal life with his medical life, but at the same time, we cannot let someone else suffer. I think if we did a better job of training all healthcare professionals about a balanced life and incorporated this training into all of our learning systems, then we would all benefit greatly. I believe learning the psychology of healing should be just as important as learning anatomy or pathology. Apparently, so does Dr. Remen.

There is no doubt in my mind that if a patient remains in a state of fear, it's very difficult for him to get well or healed. The physician/patient connection is very important to dissipating that fear, and without trust between the two, the best results can rarely be achieved. I would love to work with other professionals to come up with a way to do a short and basic psychological profile of the patient prior to initiating care. That basic psychological profile would be an extremely helpful tool for the physicians and healthcare workers who communicate with that patient. In my clinic setting now, I can easily imagine doing a short profile for a patient coming in for an initial or a subspecialty visit. The profile could be put on his electronic medical record, and knowing if someone was more analytically based or emotionally based might very well change how communication would transpire. If the physician or healthcare professional were trained about how to approach different personality types, this would further strengthen the connection between the healer and the patient. A physician could put his ego aside when he was asked twenty questions, knowing that a person with an analytical background can't help but be who he is and needs facts to get to a comfort level where he can accept his care. A person with a "take action" personality, in contrast, wouldn't need a lot of explanation other than the basic facts; he just wants to get the job done.

Our patients need to be able to trust their caregiver so they can stay in a positive place without fear and achieve maximum healing. If we as professionals simply do our job, that will help tremendously. But the patient has a role as well. It begins with fully realizing the importance of trust and connection with his caregiver. If patients have concerns about their care, then they should ask questions or get another opinion. Today patients have greater access to information about a physician than ever before. Most medical groups now place a lot of emphasis on patient satisfaction. Patients many times receive questionnaires after their visit about their experience with the caregiver or facility. Those evaluations of the physician and the clinical setting are becoming more transparent for all patients to see and play an important role in the peer review of physicians in their medical groups as well as the facilities rendering care. If a patient knew that his physician had high patient satisfaction scores, trust could form more easily. Patients need to be vigilant as they try to find the physician who can give them the best care, and the physicians need to have their feet held to the fire to provide that great care.

There are other ways patients can look for excellent physicians they can connect with. Simple tools online like Yelp can sometimes provide excellent information, biased or unbiased, similar to what Trip Advisor provides for restaurants or hotels. The information may not always be valid, but at least one can look for red flags. Medical group websites are now filled with lots of information about medical groups and their providers. If you go to the website for my medical group, www.pamf.org, you can see my areas of expertise, my resume that includes my training, my practice experience, and maybe even a video of me. I do believe video profiles can be very helpful for the patient. If the profiles are less than two minutes, most people will actually watch them. In fact, my wife and oldest son have a video production company that creates video profiles for businesses and different types of professionals. I can't tell you how many people have come to see me who have told me the reason they came to me was because of that video profile. All this information can help the patient choose the physician he can connect with best. Patients do have a choice about who takes care of them, and the more they feel they can connect with their physician, the better care they'll get.

Communication and education are imperative to excellent patient care—not just between the physician and the patient, but among all members of the patient's healthcare team. Treatment choices depend on a number of factors, such as age, current health, activity level, and personality. It takes communication with other specialist to agree on what steps are imperative for success. Just because I think someone needs surgical care for a problem doesn't mean that he is medically or psychologically ready. The patient needs to be cleared medically for the procedure and his medical after care is just as important as the preparation. For me, the goal is excellence of care, which requires a concerted effort with everybody playing their part. Of course, the patient plays a part, too, and it's our job to educate patients so they know what to expect and how to proceed. The ultimate end is to restore quality of life with everybody working together as a team.

TRANSFORMING OUR HEALTHCARE SYSTEM

As we think about changing our healthcare system, we must poll every individual who affects the environment we offer our patients. We can't afford to overlook any aspect of what it takes to create a positive, healing environment and how to steer away from one that is negative. Multidisciplinary seminars, workshops, and open forums with patients and healers can direct the process and accelerate the mission. Honestly sharing our experiences by letting go of our ego when we do not hit our mark with our care is helpful to ourselves, others, and the care of the patient. I would charge every healing professional to work together to advance our network of healing skills—over personal prestige, comfort, or fortune.

When I started my journey in medicine, I had an idealistic picture of what it was all about. That visionary picture still exists in my mind. I see the unselfish collaboration of experts in their field of training as they help heal those in need and bring health and dignity to patients' lives. I've spent my career taking care of my patients as if they were my family or friends. I've had colleagues, such as my good friend, mentor, and former partner David, who have also upheld this superior standard of care.

David was another hand and upper extremity surgeon who worked with me as one of my partners in San Diego, and we did many cases together and shared many ideas over almost three decades. We discussed problems that arose and how to best affect our cures—all without ego, always prioritizing the patient's best interest. We would assist each other in surgery, and it was the ultimate surgical experience. Two heads are better than one, and nothing could be better than having the perfect assistant. When you connect and work with people on that level, you can't help but attain an excellent result; the experience is second to none. I wish we all were open to working together in a collaborative environment. When

I think about my time working with David, I can't help but smile at his integrity, friendship, and guidance. His humility and professionalism warms my heart.

Related to that vision, I would like to see something like a patient advocate system integrated into our healthcare system. In the past, the primary care physician would follow the patient to the hospital and be at his side through anything that transpired involving his health. That still happens to some degree, but in many ways healthcare today is more disjointed. Patients often see multiple specialists, and sometimes the communication between all the specialists is less than satisfactory. They often lack a "quarterback" to coordinate their care. When a patient or his family doesn't fully understand all the parameters of an illness, they feel fearful and uncertain about what to do.

I suggest a system where a patient advocate follows a patient from start to finish and helps coordinate information and presents it to the patient and his family in a way that brings comfort and understanding. Then, hopefully, questions would be answered and care could proceed in a positive manner.

Once we developed the system, we could train experienced professionals for this role. It could be incorporated into the insurance system, and even though there would be costs associated with it, it should greatly aid in saving costs per patient, reducing the number of tests and consultations needed to address the uncertainty of a condition. I believe there are plenty of experienced, compassionate, and understanding providers who may be at the end of their career or who only want to work part-time. They would be perfect to be trained for a role such as this.

I would also like to see us do a much better job at integrating more holistic approaches to healthcare for the best healing results. I strongly believe that energy healing may play a major role in the future of medicine, and I understand the importance of alternative treatment programs, such as meditation, to help bring down one's fear and stress level and keep somebody in a positive energy state. I've always believed in "different strokes for different folks." What works for one person may not work for another, and everybody should have the opportunity to have his treatment tailored to what works for him. For example, my wife would welcome any alternative treatment to help any ill that comes her way if it meant not having to take pills or undergo surgery. Others might quickly want to "cut to the chase."

It's way past due for those of us trained in Western-based medicine to start working together in an open forum with Eastern medical practitioners, trying to combine the best of what they do with our own best practices. A group of neuroscientists get together once a year with the Dalai Lama to work together on this very thing. There is no better time than today to get the ball rolling, and I would challenge you to meet, discuss, and problem solve together. I am open to joining all those who are willing and interested to make this idea a healthcare reality.

In addition to learning preventative techniques from alternative medicine, the best preventative techniques are also the simplest: diet and exercise. Even though I'm not a nutritional expert, there's no doubt that a healthy lifestyle with a balanced diet, appropriate for one's medical issues, is great for one's health. Also, as we grow older, we will lose flexibility and strength, so it's very important to exercise regularly. I am a daily exerciser, and it helps me keep my stress levels minimal, keep my body energetic, and keep my mind positive. Exercise helps keeps one energized and in good health, as long as you don't take it to the extreme and injure yourself. Yoga combines the best of all worlds, keeping one centered, flexible, and energized. And varying your activity on a regular basis—or cross-training, as it's known in the fitness world—helps you not only minimize injuries but stay motivated and avoid boredom. If you invest more in your nutritional, physical, and emotional health, then if you become ill, you're almost assured of healing more quickly.

With a strong connection between healthcare professionals and their patients and an increased understanding of the Eastern and Western healing tools available to us, we could then attack the next challenges in healthcare: the obstacles created by the insurance, legal, and pharmaceutical industry.

First, it is time for all of us to attack the insurance industry. The Obamacare initiatives have definitely helped change some of our system's inadequacies, such as the availability of healthcare for all, and have helped to rid the exclusion of pre-existing conditions. What it hasn't done is help bring those healthcare costs down. Insurance costs for many are higher than ever, with deductibles much higher than before Obamacare. As a result of these high deductibles, people are not receiving the preventative care and evaluations they need, and I believe people's health will suffer as a result. Insurance companies are making more money than ever by raising their deductibles from five hundred dollars to five thousand, for example, to cover care for those who are uninsured or have pre-existing conditions. It is time for all of us, again, to lobby our politicians in Congress to come up with a federally based insurance plan that is truly affordable and available to all, so that insurance companies will have to reduce their deductibles and premiums to an acceptable level.

Regarding the legal system, a stronger, more powerful peer review within medical groups, hospitals, and subspecialty groups would help us to do our own house cleaning for those providers who aren't working at the optimal standard of care. As I mentioned previously, my medical group has its own risk management team that reviews and resolves issues that arise from physician or patient complaints, we are self-insured for malpractice, and we have our own legal team. If we could follow our practice's model on a widespread level, malpractice premiums would go down, as well as overall medical costs.

Finally, the pharmaceutical lobby has kept the costs of drugs frustratingly high here in the United States. Many people try to get their medications from Canada, Mexico, or even overseas, where costs for the same drugs are much lower. I get very upset when I hear countless stories about patients who can't get the medications they need for their care. Let's take, for example, someone who has cancer and needs a three-drug chemotherapy regimen to achieve maximal results and hopefully a cure. Due to the high costs of these drugs, sometimes the patient cannot afford medication for the treatment or the insurance company will not pay for the whole drug regimen. As a result, the patient can't get the care he needs for his best chance for a cure. How despicable is that? Everybody deserves the same best chance for maximum healing. It's time to stop this craziness and bring these costs down so that necessary medications are affordable for all, regardless of age, insurance, or condition. It's time for the healthcare provider and the patient to work in concert politically to bring down this pharmaceutical lobby and afford all of us the best care we can get.

Our healthcare system, with some economic and visionary changes, has the potential to extend our healing potential to a place never imagined. Researchers who delve into stem cells and alternative healing pathways will help lead the way. A true understanding of quantum physics and the energy of healing may further enlighten us in an alternative approach to health and illness. The possibilities are endless and, unless constrained, give us a hope for an exciting future.

We are all blessed to be in this wonderful world, and I'm filled with gratitude for the life that has been bestowed upon me and the incredible people I get to treat and work with. In my life and practice, it is very important to me to come from a loving place and help take people from a place of fear, ego, and greed to a place of trust and compassion. My ultimate goal is to get people to a place of positive energy, which is healing in and of itself. To reach this goal, there are things that we need to maintain as well as things we need to change. I believe that allied healthcare providers, Eastern and Western medical practitioners, and patients all working together can help bring about transformational change. The result would be happier and healthier lives for all.

I challenge you to join the movement and help make this vision our reality. Visit www.thecuttingedgeofcompassion.com

or www.drbarryrose.com and get in touch, so we can benefit from your expertise and interests. Your input and commitment are just what we need to start the ball rolling. Together, we can transform healthcare!

ACKNOWLEDGEMENTS

This book has been impacted by many amazing people in my life.

I want to thank and dedicate this book to my wife, Rose, whose love, devotion, and wisdom have been a great source of strength. Her creativity, intuition, and insight have inspired me to go after my dreams and have taken me to an awareness I never could have imagined. She is one of my greatest teachers and a blessing.

I also want to thank my patients who have taught me so much about life and how to truly care and heal.

I treasure the mentors in my life, especially Bernard Brown and David Subin MD, who have been pillars of integrity. Sharing life with them has been a blessing. This book is a result of a promise to my dear friend Bernard before his passing.

I want to thank my five loving children: Michael, Phillip, Jessica, Justin, and Jake, who have been blessings and a great source of my joy. They have been understanding and patient throughout decades of having a parent as a dedicated healer.

My editor, Amanda Rooker, shares my healing passion and has been invaluable in helping steer me in the right direction as a new author.

Last but not least, as our work continues today, I must thank my devoted colleagues who work with me compassionately to help others heal.

ABOUT THE AUTHOR

Barry Rose MD is an orthopedic surgeon who was born in 1953 and raised in Kansas City. He attended the University of Kansas for undergraduate studies and completed medical school, his internship, and his residency at the University of Kansas Medical Center. He also completed a hand/upper extremity fellowship at the University of California, San Diego. He is currently the chief of orthopedics and the surgical division head for the Alameda division of the Palo Alto Foundation Medical Group. Dr. Rose is passionate about his patients and the future of healthcare. He lives in San Francisco with his wife Rose.